South University Library
Richmond Campus
2151 Old Brick Road
Glen Allen, Va 23060

Y0-AKS-292

FEB 20 2018

CARDIOLOGY RESEARCH AND CLINICAL DEVELOPMENTS

CARDIOVASCULAR SYSTEM

ANATOMY AND PHYSIOLOGY, SHORT AND LONG-TERM EFFECTS OF EXERCISE AND ABNORMALITIES

CARDIOLOGY RESEARCH AND CLINICAL DEVELOPMENTS

Additional books in this series can be found on Nova's website under the Series tab.

Additional e-books in this series can be found on Nova's website under the e-book tab.

CARDIOLOGY RESEARCH AND CLINICAL DEVELOPMENTS

CARDIOVASCULAR SYSTEM

ANATOMY AND PHYSIOLOGY, SHORT AND LONG-TERM EFFECTS OF EXERCISE AND ABNORMALITIES

MARK E. OBERFIELD
AND
THOMAS A. SPEISER
EDITORS

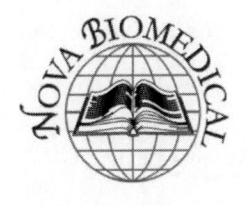

New York

Copyright © 2014 by Nova Science Publishers, Inc.

All rights reserved. No part of this book may be reproduced, stored in a retrieval system or transmitted in any form or by any means: electronic, electrostatic, magnetic, tape, mechanical photocopying, recording or otherwise without the written permission of the Publisher.

For permission to use material from this book please contact us:
Telephone 631-231-7269; Fax 631-231-8175
Web Site: http://www.novapublishers.com

NOTICE TO THE READER

The Publisher has taken reasonable care in the preparation of this book, but makes no expressed or implied warranty of any kind and assumes no responsibility for any errors or omissions. No liability is assumed for incidental or consequential damages in connection with or arising out of information contained in this book. The Publisher shall not be liable for any special, consequential, or exemplary damages resulting, in whole or in part, from the readers' use of, or reliance upon, this material. Any parts of this book based on government reports are so indicated and copyright is claimed for those parts to the extent applicable to compilations of such works.

Independent verification should be sought for any data, advice or recommendations contained in this book. In addition, no responsibility is assumed by the publisher for any injury and/or damage to persons or property arising from any methods, products, instructions, ideas or otherwise contained in this publication.

This publication is designed to provide accurate and authoritative information with regard to the subject matter covered herein. It is sold with the clear understanding that the Publisher is not engaged in rendering legal or any other professional services. If legal or any other expert assistance is required, the services of a competent person should be sought. FROM A DECLARATION OF PARTICIPANTS JOINTLY ADOPTED BY A COMMITTEE OF THE AMERICAN BAR ASSOCIATION AND A COMMITTEE OF PUBLISHERS.

Additional color graphics may be available in the e-book version of this book.

Library of Congress Cataloging-in-Publication Data

ISBN: 978-1-62948-308-5

Library of Congress Control Number: 2013950462

Published by Nova Science Publishers, Inc. † New York

Contents

Preface		vii
Chapter 1	Erythropoietin: Cell Signaling and Diseases *Zhao Zhong Chong*	1
Chapter 2	Cardiovascular Morbidities in Rheumatoid Arthritis: Effects of Exercise on Cardiac Autonomic Function *D. C. Janse van Rensburg, A. Jansen van Rensburg, C. C. Grant, J. A. Ker and L. Fletcher*	51
Chapter 3	Heart Rate Variability (HRV) Assessment of Physical Training Effects on Autonomic Cardiac Control *C. C. Grant, D. C. Janse van Rensburg, P. Sandroni and L. Fletcher*	79
Chapter 4	Autonomic Cardiovascular Control: Measurement and the Effects of Exercise *C. C. Grant, D. C. Janse van Rensburg, P. Sandroni and L. Fletcher*	101
Chapter 5	Endoplasmic Reticulum Stress in Cardiovascular Disease *Dukgyu Lee and Marek Michalak*	123

Chapter 6	Renal Sympathetic Denervation for Resistant Hypertension: Rationale and Results *Tushar Sharma, Rishi Talwar,* *Reza Khosravani Goshtaseb* *and Anjay Rastogi*	**141**
Index		**159**

Preface

The essential components of the human cardiovascular system are the heart, blood, and blood vessels. It includes: pulmonary circulation, a "loop" through the lungs where blood is oxygenated; and systemic circulation, a "loop" through the rest of the body to provide oxygenated blood. In this book, the authors present topical research in the study of the cardiovascular system and its anatomy and physiology, short and long-term effects of exercise and abnormalities. Topics discussed include erythropoietin cell signaling and diseases; cardiovascular morbidities in rheumatoid arthritis and the effects of exercise on cardiac autonomic function; heart rate variability (HRV) assessment of physical training effects on autonomic cardiac control; endoplasmic reticulum stress in cardiovascular disease; and renal sympathetic denervation for resistant hypertension.

Chapter 1 – As a hematopoietic growth factor, erythropoietin (EPO) and its receptor (EPOR) are expressed in many tissues throughout the human body in addition to erythroid cells. Consequently, the biological activity of EPO has been extended to cardiovascular, neurovascular, and many other systems. EPO is capable of modulating multiple cellular signal transduction pathways to formulate its biological functions.

Initially, EPO binds EPOR to activate the Janus-tyrosine kinase 2 (Jak2) protein followed by activation of protein kinase B (Akt), signal transducer and activators of transcription 5, mitogen-activated protein kinases, mammalian target of rapamycin, protein tyrosine phosphatases, Wnt1, and nuclear factor κB, through which EPO intervene both the physiological and pathological functions. As a result, the efficacy of EPO has been tested in cardiovascular diseases and neurodegenerative diseases. To systemic elucidate the function of EPO and EPO-mediated cell signaling pathways will allow us to reveal the therapeutic potential of EPO in diseases beyond anemia and establish the foundation for the development of therapeutic strategies through application of EPO against these diseases.

Chapter 2 – Rheumatoid Arthritis (RA) is a chronic, inflammatory disease of unknown cause and primarily considered a disease of the joints. However, a variety of extra-articular manifestations including cardiovascular (CV) involvement are well recognized. There is a growing body of literature supporting the evidence for excess cardiovascular risk in patients with RA. Possible etiopathogenesis include conventional risk factors (hypertension, abnormal body mass index, smoking, etc.), accelerated atherosclerosis i.e., due to inflammation (measured by high-sensitivity C-reactive protein (CRP) and autonomic dysfunction (either by increased disrhythmogenic potential or by neuronal pathways modulating inflammation). The autonomic nervous system is one of a variety of neuronal pathways implicated in modifying inflammation. Abnormal autonomic function is characterized by decreased heart rate variability (HRV).This may induce an increased disrhytmogenic potential. Exercise has been identified as one of the most important behavioural strategies for cardiovascular disease prevention and sedentary individuals (like RA sufferers) will benefit by even a small increase in physical activity. Many studies in non-RA groups demonstrated that exercise will improve autonomic function, as measured by HRV. The aim of this chapter is to describe the cardiac involvement in RA and to discuss the data available on the effects of exercise in RA. This will be followed by a description of an exercise intervention and the cardiovascular effects reported in a group of South African female RA sufferers. The chapter will conclude with recommendations for future research.

Chapter 3 – This Chapter reports the effects of a standardised, intensive physical training programme (energy expenditure: 8485 kJ/day) on autonomic cardiac control of a large group of healthy participants (N=154). It was hypothesized that results of exercise induced changes on the autonomic nervous system (ANS) are dependent on the body position and should be assessed not only in the resting position. Heart rate variability (HRV) recordings were made in the supine, rising and standing positions.

Analytical techniques used were time domain, frequency domain and non-linear (Poincaré) analysis.

The results of this study, for the supine position, showed an increase in resting vagal control of the heart, and a general increase in HRV by exercise programs. It also showed, with the aid of deductive reasoning, that lower post-exercise heart rate may result, not only from the exercise-induced increase in vagal activity, but that a decrease in sympathetic control of the heart contribute to it. The exercise intervention increased both vagal and sympathetic variation during rising, without redistribution of the spectral frequency component. After the intervention, sympathetic activity was increased, not only during rising, but also during the standing period. When the influence of the exercise intervention on the orthostatic response was assessed as the difference between the stationary standing period and supine, the exercise-improved orthostatic response was indicated as a, predominantly, increase in sympathetic control. The work from this study thus showed that measurement of the influence of exercise on ANS functioning are dependent on the body position and assessments should be done, not only in the resting position, but also during standing and during an orthostatic stressor.

Chapter 4 – Heart rate variability (HRV) analysis is a popular tool for the assessment of autonomic cardiac control. These measurements are increasingly employed in studies ranging from investigations of central autonomic regulation; to studies exploring the link between psychological processes and physiological functioning; to the indication of ANS activity in response to exercise, training and overtraining. Many publications elaborate on the effect of exercise on HRV and by implication on cardiac functioning. However, results on the effects of exercise on the autonomic control of the heart are often contradictory and incomplete in the normal population and in disease. In order to understand and employ the effects of exercise in patients with cardiovascular disorders it is of primary importance that agreement should be reached on the effects of exercise in the normal and healthy population.

In this chapter, a selection of older and more recent publications, investigating autonomic training effects as measured by cardiovascular variability indicators, are summarized. Reasons for heterogeneous results are identified and discussed. The chapter concludes with specific recommendations for future research.

Chapter 5 – The endoplasmic reticulum (ER), an elaborate network of membrane, is the cellular organelle supporting diverse cellular functions: protein synthesis and folding, synthesis of phospholipids and steroids, and regulation of calcium homeostasis. Environmental stimuli such as oxidative stress and ischemic insult, or the accumulation of unfolded and/or misfolded protein cause ER stress; as a result, ER stress activates the unfolded protein response (UPR) to deal with a disruption of ER homeostasis. In the cardiovascular system, ER stress is linked to the pathologic states include ischemia, pressure overload, hypertension, atherosclerosis, hypertrophy, dilated cardiomyopathy, and heart failure. The UPR process is composed of a group of signal transduction pathways that improve the accumulation of unfolded protein by inhibiting protein translation, induction of ER chaperones, and accelerating the degradation of unfolded proteins. The UPR is an adaptive response to cope with ER stress but, if unresolved, it can lead to apoptotic cell death. Therefore, the development of therapeutic interventions that target molecules of the UPR signaling pathway and ameliorate ER stress will be convincing strategies to treat cardiovascular disease and other related disorders. In this chapter, the authors will discuss the recent progress in understanding the UPR pathway in cardiovascular disease and its related healing potential.

Chapter 6 – Hypertension is a significant global cause of morbidity and mortality, affecting no less than 1 billion people worldwide. In the United States, it affects more than 1 in 3 individuals, and almost 2 in 3 individuals above age 65. Despite the use of multiple medications, a huge number of patients don't reach their desired clinical target. Historically, over activation of sympathetic nervous system has been considered as playing a part in the pathogenesis of essential hypertension, and the relation has been made clearer by the use of techniques like microneurography and noradrenaline spill-over measurements. Kidneys have been found to be of an importance cause of this sympathetic over activity. Based on this, a novel technique of renal sympathetic denervation has been developed to treat resistant hypertension. The results so far have been encouraging and it certainly deserves further research. This review article discusses the burden of hypertension, the evidence of sympathetic overdrive playing a role in its etiology, the role of kidneys and the rationale behind renal denervation. It further sheds light on the results achieved, the problems faced and the weaknesses with each study done. In the end, it focuses on the prospects of his technique and realms for future research.

In: Cardiovascular System
Editors: M. Oberfield and Th. Speiser

ISBN: 978-1-62948-308-5
© 2014 Nova Science Publishers, Inc.

Chapter 1

Erythropoietin: Cell Signaling and Diseases

Zhao Zhong Chong*
Department of Neurology and Neurosciences, Cancer Center,
New Jersey Medical School, University of Medicine and
Dentistry of New Jersey, Newark, New Jersey, US
Institute of Materia Medica, Shandong Academy of
Medical Sciences, Jinan, China

Abstract

As a hematopoietic growth factor, erythropoietin (EPO) and its receptor (EPOR) are expressed in many tissues throughout the human body in addition to erythroid cells. Consequently, the biological activity of EPO has been extended to cardiovascular, neurovascular, and many other systems. EPO is capable of modulating multiple cellular signal transduction pathways to formulate its biological functions.

Initially, EPO binds EPOR to activate the Janus-tyrosine kinase 2 (Jak2) protein followed by activation of protein kinase B (Akt), signal transducer and activators of transcription 5, mitogen-activated protein kinases, mammalian target of rapamycin, protein tyrosine phosphatases,

---

* Corresponding author: Zhao Zhong Chong, MD, PhD, Department of Neurology and Neurosciences, Cancer Center, F-1222, UMDNJ – New Jersey Medical School, 205 South Orange Avenue, Newark, NJ 07103. Tel: 973-972-0548; E-mail: zzchong@yahoo.com.

Wnt1, and nuclear factor κB, through which EPO intervene both the physiological and pathological functions. As a result, the efficacy of EPO has been tested in cardiovascular diseases and neurodegenerative diseases. To systemic elucidate the function of EPO and EPO-mediated cell signaling pathways will allow us to reveal the therapeutic potential of EPO in diseases beyond anemia and establish the foundation for the development of therapeutic strategies through application of EPO against these diseases.

Historic Aspect of EPO

In 1906, Paul Carnot, a professor of the University of Paris, France, and his assistant, Clotilde Deflandre, conducted an experiment in which they injected plasma withdrawn from rabbits subject to bloodletting into normal rabbits, which resulted in a dramatic increase in immature red blood cells in recipients. Based on the breaking outcome, they proposed that a substance in the blood regulates the erythropoiesis and named it as hemopoietine (Carnot and DeFlandre 1906). Several investigators continued to study in this field to confirm the hypothesis and positive results emerged again after twenty-six years of efforts. Sandor found that serum from rabbits subjected to hypoxia caused reticulocytosis in the recipients in 1932 (Sandor 1932), the phenomenon of reticulocytosis was further revealed in rabbits that received serum from bloodletting rabbits (Hiort 1936; Krumdieck 1943). In 1948, Eve Bonsdorff and Eve Jalavisto renamed hemopoietine as erythropoietin (EPO) (Bonsdorff and Jalavisto 1948), since the hormone initially increase the production of red blood cells.

To clarify the molecular structure and get insight into the mystery of EPO, the key is to isolate and purify EPO. Dr. Eugene Goldwasser and his colleagues from University of Chicago worked on purification of EPO for over 20 years and invented a seven-step procedure of purification and successfully isolated eight milligram of EPO from 2550 liters of urine from patients with aplastic anemia in 1977 (Miyake et al. 1977). The success should also ascribe to Dr. Takaji Mijake from Kumamoto University in Japan who had collected and concentrated the urine and sent to Goodwasser on Christmas day in 1975. Two years later, fetal liver, not the kidney, was found as the primarily site to produce EPO in sheep (Zanjani et al. 1977).

Thanks to the purified EPO sample given by Goodwasser, Amgen (Applied Molecular Genetics at that time) cloned human EPO gene in 1985

(Lin et al. 1985), paving the way to gross production and clinical application of human recombinant EPO.

Soon later, Amgen began the clinical trial of EPO for anemia and found that EPO is effective in the treatment of anemia with end stage renal failure (Eschbach et al. 1987; Winearls et al. 1986). Amgen marketed its first EPO product Epogen in 1989, the profit of which help the Amgen grow to be one of world top pharmaceutical companies.

Structural Aspect of EPO

Human EPO, a 30.4 kDa glycoprotein, is the encoding product of EPO gene. The EPO gene is located on chromosome 7, exists as a single copy in a 5.4 kb region of the genomic DNA, and encodes a polypeptide chain containing 193 amino acids (Jacobs et al. 1985). During secretion of EPO, a 166 amino acid peptide is initially generated following the cleavage of a 27 amino acid hydrophobic secretory leader at the amino-terminal (Imai et al. 1990).

In addition, a carboxy-terminal arginine in position 166 is removed both in mature human and recombinant human EPO (Imai et al. 1990). Consequently, the circulatory mature protein of EPO is a 165 amino acid peptide.

Over 40% of molecular weight of EPO is attributable to its carbohydrates content. EPO contains four glycosylated chains including three N-linked and one O-linked acidic oligosaccharide side chains. N-linked glycosylation sites occur at the positions 24, 38, and 83 of aspartyl residues, while the O-linked glycosylation site is at serine 126.

Three N-glycan chains of human EPO consist of the tetra-antennary structure with or without N-acetyllactosamine repeating units (Tsuda et al. 1988). The O-linked sugar chain is composed of Gal-GalNAc and sialic acids (Sasaki et al. 1987). The production and secretion of the mature EPO also relies upon the integrity of the N- and O-linked chains.

The glycosylated chains are important for the biological activity of EPO and can protect EPO from oxygen radical degradation. The carbohydrate chains stabilize human EPO (Toyoda et al. 2000) and the oligosaccharides in EPO may protect the protein from oxygen radical activity (Uchida et al. 1997). The N-glycosylated chains are believed to contribute to the thermal stability of EPO (Tsuda et al. 1988).

In addition, the N- and O-linked chains may be necessary for the production and secretion of the mature EPO (Krantz 1991). Replacement of asparagines 38 and 83 by glutamate or serine 126 by glycine can decrease the production and secretion of EPO (Dube et al. 1988).

The presence of the carbohydrates also is important in the control of the metabolism of EPO, since EPO molecules with high sialic acid content can be easily cleared by the body through specific binding in the liver (Tsuda et al. 1988).

In addition, the biological activity of EPO also relies upon two disulfide bonds formed between cysteines at positions 7 and 160 and at positions 29 and 33. The requirement of these disulfide bridges has been demonstrated by the evidence that reduction of these bonds results in the loss of the biologic activity of EPO. Alkylation of the sulfhydryl groups results in irreversible loss of the biological activity of EPO. Re-oxidization of EPO after reduction by guanidine restores eighty-five percent of the biological activity of EPO (Wang et al. 1985). Cysteine 33 replacement with proline also reduces the biological function of EPO.

EPO Expression throughout the Body

Endogenous EPO is initially produced in the fetal liver, but is subsequently shifted to the kidney in the adult. Human liver is the primary site of EPO gene expression both in fetal and neonatal period of life (Dame et al. 1998). The identification of the kidney as the producing site of EPO is primarily attributable to the work of Leon Jacobson and his colleagues who found that nephrectomised rats fail to increase plasma EPO in response to hypoxia (Jacobson et al. 1957). This hypothesis was supported by the followed work demonstrating an increased EPO level in the perfusates of isolated kidneys perfused with blood of reduced oxygen tension (Fisher and Birdwell 1961; Kuratowska et al. 1961). Further study indicates that kidney cortex is the major site to produce EPO (Jelkmann and Bauer 1981) and the immunoreactivity of EPO is revealed in peritubular endothelial cells of the anemic mouse kidney (Suzuki and Sasaki 1990) and peritubular fibroblasts of the rat kidney cortex (Bachmann and Weber 1993).

In addition to the kidney and liver, other organs including bone marrow, vascular smooth muscle, spleen, reproductive organs (uterus, oviduct, placenta, ovary, testis) have been identified to secrete EPO (Chong et al. 2002b; Fisher 2003). At cellular level, the kidney peritubular interstitial cells, Kuffer cells, hepatocytes, peripheral endothelial cells (ECs), muscle cells, enterocytes, and insulin-producing cells are responsible for EPO production in different tissues (Anagnostou et al. 1994; Chong et al. 2002a; Chong et al. 2002b; Ribatti et al. 1999).

Since astrocytes were found to produce EPO (Masuda et al. 1994) and the expression of EPOR was found on neuronal cells (Masuda et al. 1993) in the central nervous system (CNS), the investigations of biological function of EPO in the CNS have attracted great interest. Since then, both EPO and the EPOR have been found to functionally express in the nervous system of rodents, primates, and humans.

In the mouse brain, EPO is present in the hippocampus, capsula interna, cortex, and midbrain areas (Digicaylioglu et al. 1995). In the rat brain, the expression of EPO and EPOR has been found in neurons, astrocytes, and ECs (Chong et al. 2003a; Masuda et al. 1994).

In cultured cortical neurons of rats, the expression of EPOR has been demonstrated by immunostaining and reverse transcription-polymerase chain reaction (Morishita et al. 1997). Immunocytochemical staining has revealed the expression of EPO and the EPOR in rat hippocampal neurons (Chong et al. 2002b; Chong et al. 2003b). In primates, mRNA of EPO and the EPOR gene are present in the hippocampus, amygdala, and temporal cortex of the brain (Marti et al. 1996).

In the human brain, EPO and the EPOR are present in both astrocytes and neurons (Juul et al. 1999). There is an elevated level of EPO in the cerebrospinal fluid during embryogenesis that is gradually reduced after birth, but is still kept at a low level throughout the adulthood (Marti et al. 1997; Velly et al. 2010). Accumulating work has documented the presence of the EPOR on neurons, microglia, astrocytes, cerebral ECs, and on myelin sheaths in human peripheral nerves (Chong et al. 2003b; Genc et al. 2004; Marti 2004; Morishita et al. 1997). The production of EPO and the expression of the EPOR in brain tissue strongly suggest a significant role of EPO in the CNS.

EPO Production and Oxygen Tension

In response to hypoxia, the plasma EPO level can be increased up to 1000 fold above the normal level. It is the tissue oxygen tension, neither the number of red blood cells, nor the level of hemoglobin, that critically regulates EPO production and erythropoiesis. Low oxygen tension induced expression of EPO is dependent on hypoxia-inducible factor (HIF-1).

HIF-1 is a basic helix–loop–helix heterodimeric transcription factor containing two subunits, HIF-1α and HIF-1β. HIF-1α is a 120-kDa oxygen-labile subunit that is degraded through the ubiquitin-proteasome pathway under normoxic conditions (Huang et al. 1998).

Three HIF-α isoforms have been identified as HIF-1α, HIF-2α, and HIF-3α. HIF-1α is the most widely expressed isoform in mammalian cells. HIF-1β is constitutively expressed in the nucleus. HIF-1β is a 91–94 kDa protein that is characterized as aryl hydrocarbon receptor nuclear translocator (ARNT) (Hoffman et al. 1991) and also has three HIF-β isoforms named as HIF-1β/ARNT1, ARNT2, and ARNT3.

Oxygen availability activates hydroxylases that are responsible for the regulation of HIF-α. During normoxia, the prolyl hydroxylation of HIF-α within the oxygen dependent degradation domain facilitates the binding of von Hippel-Lindau protein (pVHL) to HIF-α, leading to ubiquitylation and proteasomal degradation of HIF-α (Ivan et al. 2001). pVHL acts as the recognition component of a ubiquitin E3 ligase complex which binds HIF-α (Jaakkola et al. 2001). Factor-inhibiting HIF-1 (FIH-1), a specific asparaginyl hydroxylase, induced the asparaginyl hydroxylation of HIF-α in the C-terminal transactivation domain during normoxia results in the blockade of its interaction with transcriptional coactivator p300/ CREB binding protein (CBP) (Lando et al. 2002).

During hypoxia, the hydroxylases are inactivated and HIF-α is stabilized, translocates to the nucleus, and heterodimerizes with HIF-β to form a stable HIF-1 complex to induce transcription of genes that are involved in erythropoiesis and angiogenesis. Specifically, the HIF complex binds to the conserved sequence (5′RCGTG3′) near the 5′ end of the hypoxia-responsive enhancer of the EPO gene to up-regulate EPO gene transcription (Bunn et al. 1998) (Figure 1). Further study indicates that HIF-2α is responsible for hypoxia-induced EPO expression in the hapatoma cells and the human neuroblastoma cells (Warnecke et al. 2004).

The hepatic nuclear factor-4 (HNF-4) also plays a role in hypoxia induced EPO gene transcription. HNF-4 is constitutively expressed in kidney, liver, and other EPO-producing cells. Functional experiments indicate that HNF-4 controls the tissue-specificity of EPO gene transcription and enhances hypoxia-inducible expression of the EPO gene (Galson et al. 1995). HNF-4 is an orphan nuclear receptor that cooperates with HIF-1 and transcription coactivator p300 to form a macromolecular assembly to give maximal hypoxic induction of transcription (Bunn et al. 1998)

In the CNS, the expression of EPO is also upregulated in response to hypoxia. Hypoxia induces the upregulation of HIF-α expression in the rat brain cortex and HIF-1α was further identified in neurons, astrocytes, ependymal cells, and possibly endothelial cells (Chavez et al. 2000).

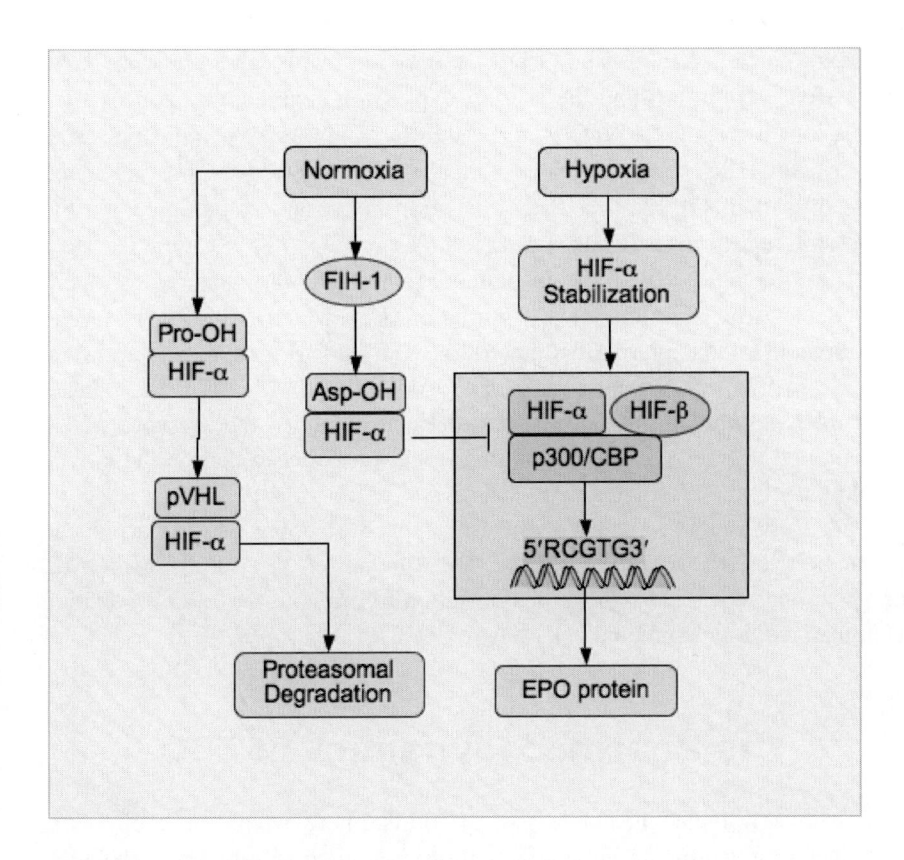

Figure 1. Hypoxia induces transcription of gene of erythropoietin (EPO) through hypoxia-inducible factor-1 (HIF-1). Under normoxic condition, the prolyl hydroxylation (Pro-OH) of HIF-1α within the oxygen dependent degradation domain promotes the binding of von Hippel-Lindau protein (pVHL) to HIF-α, leading to ubiquitylation and proteasomal degradation of HIF-α. Oxygen also keep the activation of Factor-inhibiting HIF-1 (FIH-1), a specific asparaginyl hydroxylase, to induce the asparaginyl hydroxylation of HIF-1α in the C-terminal transactivation domain during normoxia, resulting in the blockade of its interaction with transcriptional coactivator p300/ CREB binding protein (CBP). Hypoxia inactivates hydroxylases and HIF-α is stabilized, translocates to the nucleus, and heterodimerizes with HIF-β to form a stable HIF-1 complex to bind to the conserved sequence (5'RCGTG3') near the 5' end of the hypoxia-responsive enhancer of the EPO gene to up-regulate EPO gene transcription with the assistance of transcription coactivator p300/CBP.

In response to hypoxia, EPO expression is increased up to 100-fold in primary cultured mouse astrocytes (Marti et al. 1996). The EPO mRNA expression is also enhanced by hypoxia in both astrocytes and neurons (Bernaudin et al. 2000). Gene silence of HIF-1α in astrocytes abrogates hypoxia-induced VEGF and LDH expression with alteration in EPO expression; yet diminishing the HIF-2α expression significantly reduces EPO expression in response to hypoxia. In addition, Chip assay demonstrates that HIF-2α, not HIF-1α, is associated with the EPO hypoxia-response element, suggesting that HIF-2α mediates the transcriptional activation of EPO expression in astrocytes (Chavez et al. 2006).

The production of EPO in female reproductive organs is estrogen-dependent. Administration of 17β-estradiol (E$_2$), which controls the cyclic development of the uterine endometrium, can lead to a rapid and transient increase in EPO mRNA in the uterus (Yasuda et al. 1998). Hypoxia induced EPO mRNA expression in uterine tissue occurs only in the presence of E$_2$. This induction by hypoxia in the uterus is less pronounced than in the kidney (Chikuma et al. 2000). Oviduct and ovary production of EPO is also E$_2$ dependent (Masuda et al. 2000). But E2 appears to suppress hypoxia-induced production of EPO in the kidney (Mukundan et al. 2002). Moreover, progesterone, not E2, has been demonstrated to promote the EPO production in human amniotic epithelial cells (Ogawa et al. 2003).

The Pharmacodynamics of EPO

The absorption of the single-dose of 50 U/kg body weight of recombinant human EPO given by the intraperitoneal (ip) is limited with minimal elevation of serum EPO from 27 ± 3 mU/l to a plateau of 36 ± 4 mU/l at 12-24 hrs. In contrast, a peak EPO level of EPO reaches 81 ± 13 mU/l) 24 hrs after subcutaneous (sc) injection, which also increases the areas under the concentration-time curve from 0 to 24 hrs and elevates the hemoglobin level by approximately 40% over 16 weeks period (Lui et al. 1990), suggesting that administration of EPO *via* sc injection is effective way of treatment. After the subcutaneous injection of EPO, the mean absorption time is 22 ± 11 h and bioavailability is 44 ± 7% in patients under chronic haemodialysis (Brockmoller et al. 1992). The half-life of EPO after first intravenous injection is 5.4 ±1.7 hr, the volume of distribution is 70 ± 5.2 ml/kg, and the clearance is 10.1 ± 3.5 ml/h/kg.

Yet, the half-life of steady state after 3 months of continuous therapy is decreased 4.6 ± 2.8 h), but no change in mean clearance and volume of distribution is observed (Brockmoller et al. 1992).

EPO and Cellular Signaling Pathways

EPO binds to EPOR to induce a series of cellular signal transduction pathways following the activation of EPOR. The EPOR is a type 1 superfamily of cytokine receptors, which contain a common domain structure consisting of an extracellular ligand-binding domain, a transmembrane domain, and an intracellular domain. The extracellular domain is necessary for the initial binding of EPO and the intracellular domain is responsible for the transduction of intracellular signaling (Mulcahy 2001).

The intracellular domain of the EPOR contains a Box 1 motif that specifically binds to and activates Janus tyrosine kinase 2 (Jak2) by phosphorylation (Witthuhn et al. 1993). Jak2 contains a kinase domain in the carboxyl portion, a kinase-like domain, and a large amino-terminal domain that binds to the β-subunit of the EPOR at a region proximal to the Box 1 sequence (Zhao et al. 1995). EPO can prevent apoptotic neuronal injury through Jak2 phosphorylation, since transfection of cortical neurons with a biologically incompetent Jak2 construction abrogates EPO mediated protection (Digicaylioglu and Lipton 2001).

Following the activation of Jak2, EPO modulates cell survival through several downstream signals, such as phosphoinositol 3-kinase (PI3K)/Akt, signal transducer and activator of transcriptions (STATs), extracellular signal related kinase (ERK) proteins, nuclear factor-κB (NF-κB), mammalian target of rapamycin (mTOR), protein tyrosine phosphatases (PTPs), and Wnt1 (Figure 2).

EPO and PI3K/Akt

Akt, also known as protein kinase B, plays a critical role in cell survival. Activation of Akt is dependent on PI3K that consists of two subunits, a regulatory subunit (85 kDa) and a catalytic subunit (110 ka). Growth factors or cytokines can stimulate the recruitment of PI3K to the plasma membrane for activation.

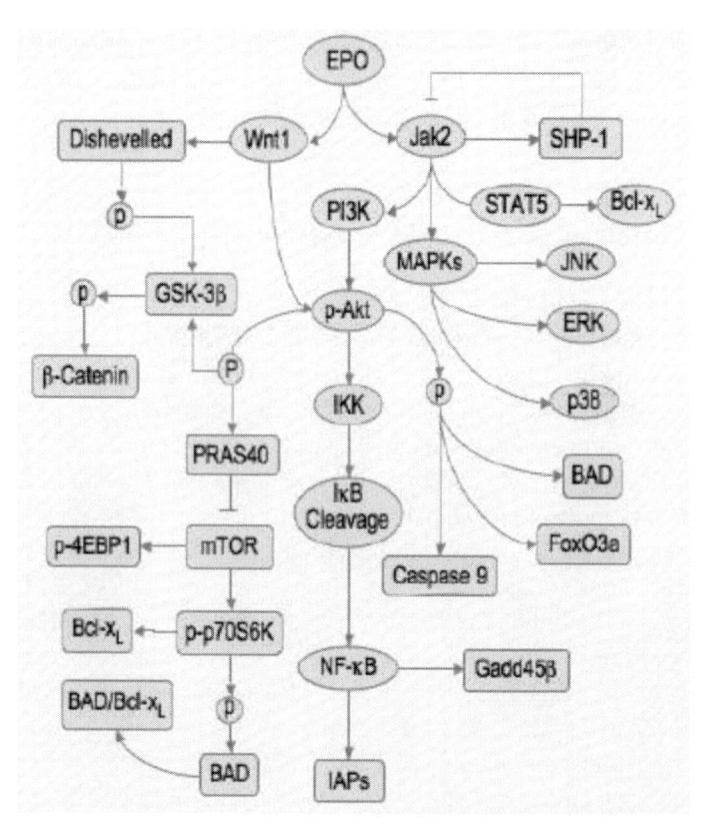

Figure 2. Erythropoietin (EPO) mediates multiple signal transduction pathways. EPO binds to its receptor (EPOR) resulting in the phosphorylation and activation of the Janus tyrosine kinase 2 (Jak2). The activated Jak2 mediates the recruitment and activation of phosphoinositol 3 kinase (PI3K)/Akt, signal transducer and activator of transcription 5 (STAT5), and extracellular signal related kinase (ERK) followed by regulation of Bcl-x_L, inhibitors of apoptotic protein (IAPs), FoxO3a, glycogen synthase kinase (GSK)-3β, Bad, I-κB kinae (IKK), nuclear factor (NF)-κB, and the growth arrest and DNA damage (Gadd) 45β. SHP-1 acts as a negative regulator of the EPOR and Jak2 activity. EPO can also regulate Wnt1, which can bind to its transmembrane receptor followed by recruitment of disheveled, the cytoplasmic bridging molecule. EPO phosphorylates glycogen synthase kinase-3β (GSK-3β) through Wnt1 to prevent β-catenin phosphorylation and promote the nuclear translocation of β-catenin to increase transcription of anti-apoptotic genes. In addition, EPO can target mammalian target of rapamycin (mTOR) to prevent apoptosis *via* phosphorylating 40 kDa proline-rich Akt1 substrate (PRAS40). Following activation of mTOR, p70 ribosomal S6 kinase (p70S6K) and eukaryotic initiation factor 4E-binding protein 1 (4EBP1) are phosphorylated. The activated p70S6K increases the expression of Bcl-x_L, phosphorylates Bad, resulting in the dissociation of Bad with Bcl-x_L and more available Bcl-x_L.

Following activation, PI3K phosphorylates phosphoinositide, phosphatidylinositide 3-phosphate (PIP), and phosphatidylinositide (3,4)-bisphosphate (PIP$_2$), producing PIP, PIP$_2$, and phosphatidylinositide (3,4,5)-triphosphate (PIP$_3$) respectively and resulting in the transition of Akt from the cytosol to the plasma membrane by the binding of Akt to PIP$_2$ and PIP$_3$ through its plectrin homology (PH) domain. Akt is subsequently phosphorylated by phosphoinositide dependent kinase (PDK) 1 and PDK2 (Chong et al. 2005b; Chong et al. 2012a; Stephens et al. 1998).

PDK1 and PDK2 phosphorylate threonine308 and serine473 of Akt respectively. PDK1 contains a C-terminal PH domain through which PIP$_3$ recruits PDK1 to the cell membrane and binds to the C-terminal hydrophobic motif (HM) domain of Akt and specifically phosphorylates Akt at threonine308. Although the phosphorylation on the residue of serine473 is necessary for the full activation of Akt, PDK1 cannot directly phosphorylate Akt on the serine473. It is PDK2 that is responsible for the phosphorylation of Akt on serine473. Several kinases have been identified to have PDK2 like activity such as intergrin-linked kinase, DNA dependent protein kinase, protein kinase C-beta (PKCβ), and mammalian target of rapamycin complex 2 (mTORC2) (Chong et al. 2012c).

EPO phosphorylates Akt through activating Jak2 and PI3K. Activation of Jak2 promotes the phosphorylation of tryrosine residues at position of 479 in the intracellular portion of the EPOR (Nguyen et al. 2001). Phosphorylation of the tyrosine of the EPOR initiates the binding of the 85-kDa regulatory subunit of PI3K, leading to the activation of 110-kDa catalytic subunit and subsequent activation of Akt.

Akt is a well-established pro-survival serine/threonine kinase that can maintain cell survival against a variety of injuries (Chong et al. 2004; Chong et al. 2006; Das et al. 2007; Matsuzaki et al. 1999; Yu et al. 2005). The downstream components of the Akt pathway include pro-apoptotic protein BAD, caspase 9, the forkhead transcription factor (FHKRL1, FoxO3a), and glycogen synthase kinase-3β (GSK3β). Akt target these signals to block the progression of apoptosis by inactivation of these proteins *via* phosphorylation.

Phosphorylation of BAD promotes its interaction with the cytosolic docking protein 14-3-3 resulting in the liberation of the anti-apoptotic protein Bcl-2/Bcl-x$_L$ (Chong et al. 2003b; Shang et al. 2012; Shen et al. 2010). The phosphorylation of FoxO3a also results in its recruitment by the 14-3-3 protein and its cytoplasmic retention, rendering it unable to regulate its target genes in the nucleus for the induction of apoptosis (Brunet et al. 1999; Chong et al. 2011; Chong et al. 2007b; Chong and Maiese 2007a; Hou et al. 2010;

Mahmud et al. 2002; Maiese 2008; Shang et al. 2009a; Shang et al. 2009b; Shang et al. 2010). Inhibition of GSK-3β activity by phosphorylation through Akt can result in its inactivation and block the induction of apoptosis (Chong et al. 2007a; Kim et al. 2008; Shang et al. 2007).

EPO and STATs

STAT proteins are latent cytosolic transcription factors and direct substrates of Janus tyrosine kinases. Activation of Jak2 results in the phosphorylation of tyrosine residues, leading to dimerization and activation of STATs. Once activated, STATs translocate to the nucleus and bind to specific DNA sequences in the promoter regions of responsive genes to lead to gene transcription. Specifically, the phosphorylation of tyrosine^{343} and tyrosine^{401} in the intracellular domain of the EPOR is responsible for activation of the two isoforms of STAT5, known as STAT5a and STAT5b, respectively (Gobert et al. 1996). In response to EPO stimulation, STAT5 can bind to the Bcl-x$_L$ promoter to induce Bcl-x$_L$ expression and prevent apoptosis (Shang et al. 2012; Socolovsky et al. 1999; Zhang et al. 2007) (Figure 2).

EPO and ERK

ERK is one of the components of the mitogen-activated protein kinases (MAPKs), which also include the c-Jun-amino terminal kinases (JNKs), and the p38 kinase. Phosphorylation of tyrosine464 on the intracellular domain of EPOR results in the activation of MAPKs. The phosphorylation of ERK has been suggested to account for the protection of EPO, since EPO application can increase the activation of ERK to protect neonatal rat brain against neurotoxicity (Dzietko et al. 2004). EPO has also been shown to attenuate the retinal neuronal cell death induced by glycosal-advanced glycation end products through both ERK and Akt activating pathways (Shen et al. 2010).

Yet, the neuroprotection of EPO appears to be independent of the activity of p38 and JNK (Jacobs-Helber et al. 2000).

EPO and NF-κB

The function of EPO has also been associated with the activation of the transcription factor NF-κB (Chong et al. 2005c; Digicaylioglu and Lipton 2001; Li et al. 2006). In resting cells, NF-κB is held captive by proteins of the IκB family and sequestered in the cytoplasm. In response to EPO, the active Akt can result in the activation of the IκB kinase (IKK) complex, which phosphorylates IκB, ensuring that it is ubiquitinated by the addition of a ubiquitin group and degraded, leading to the release of the bound NF-κB. The liberated NF-κB can then translocate to the nucleus and transcriptionally activate its target genes, (Kyriakis 2001) such as the inhibitors of apoptosis (IAP) protein family (c-IAP1, c-IAP2, and X-chromosome-linked IAP) (Zou et al. 2004), which specifically inhibit the active forms of caspase 3, caspase 7, and caspase 9 (Reed 2001).

In addition, the growth arrest and DNA damage (Gadd) 45β has been identified as a downstream target of NF-κB. The induction of Gadd45β protein by TNF-α is NF-κB dependent and responsible for the down regulation of JNK activation and apoptosis suppression (De Smaele et al. 2001) (Figure 2). EPO cannot only preserve the expression of NF-κBp65 *via* preventing its degradation by Aβ and also promote the subcellular translocation of NF-κBp65 from the cytoplasm to the nucleus to initiate anti-apoptotic gene transcription. In addition, gene silencing of NF-κBp65 by RNA interference reduces the ability of EPO to protect neurons against Aβ toxicity, suggesting that activation of NF-κB is necessary for EPO protection in the nervous system (Chong et al. 2005c).

EPO and mTOR

As a serine/threonine protein kinase, mTOR plays a central role in transcription, cytoskeletal organization, cell growth, and proliferation as well as cell survival (Chong et al. 2012c; Chong et al. 2010b; Chong et al. 2013; Zoncu et al. 2011). EPO can protect cells against apoptosis through activating mTOR.

In neurons, mTOR activation prevents oxidative stress induced apoptosis in PC12 cells and primary murine neurons (Chen et al. 2010) through phosphorylating eukaryotic initiation factor 4E-binding protein 1 (4EBP1) and p70 ribosomal S6 kinase (p70S6K) {Chen, 2010 #3183; Chen, 2010 #17}, two downstream targets of mTOR. Application of rapamycin to inhibit mTOR activation or transfection of mTORsiRNA into the cultures of microglia and neuronal cells prior to OGD significantly increases OGD-induced cell injury in microglia and neuronal cells (Chong et al. 2007b; Chong et al. 2012b; Shang et al. 2011), suggesting that mTOR activation may function to protect against ischemic injury in the CNS.

Further study indicates that EPO promotes the phosphorylation of mTOR and p70S6K, in contrast, application of rapamycin blocks EPO induced mTOR activation and attenuates the ability of EPO to prevent mitochondrial membrane depolarization, cytochrome c release from mitochondria, and subsequent induction of apoptosis in microglia during OGD, illustrating that EPO can protect microglia against ischemic injury through activating mTOR (Shang et al. 2011).

Proline-rich Akt substrate 40 kDa (PRAS40) emerges as the target for EPO to regulate the activity of mTOR. PRAS40 is a mTOR binding partner in mTOR complex 1 (mTORC1) and competitively inhibits the binding of mTOR substrates to regulatory-associated protein of mTOR (Raptor), an essential component of the complex that functions to recruit substrates of mTOR to the mTORC1 complex (Wang et al. 2007).

Phosphorylation of PRAS40 on the residue of threonine246 by Akt leads to its dissociation from mTORC1 and instead increases its binding to the cytoplasmic docking 14-3-3 protein (Nascimento et al. 2010), resulting in an increase in the activity of mTORC1. We have demonstrated that EPO promotes PRAS40 phosphorylation *via* Akt1, resulting in the dissociation of PRAS40 with mTOR and an increased binding of phosphorylated (p)-PRAS40 to cytoplasmic docking protein 14-3-3, leading to activation of mTOR with an increase in the expression of p-4EBP1 and p-p70S6K.

Moreover, gene silence of PRAS40 enhances the activity of mTOR, promotes the activation of mTOR, reduces the activation of caspase 3 and cell injury following OGD, but the regulation of PRAS40 phosphorylation by EPO is independent of EPO induced activation of ERK and STAT5 (Chong et al. 2012b).

EPO and PTPs

The cytoplasmic PTPs contain two SH2 NH_2-terminal domains to their catalytic phosphatase domain and are referred to as SHPs that are intimately involved in several cellular activities, such as cytoskeletal maintenance, cell division, and cell differentiation (Chong and Maiese 2007b; Feng et al. 1994). Of these, two particular SHP proteins known as SHP1 and SHP2 have been linked to Jak2 and play an important role in the EPO signal transduction pathways. SHP-1 can associate with EPO receptor *via* its SH2 domains by binding to the tyrosine429 residue in the cytoplasmic domain of the EPO receptor. This action prevents EPO from activating Jak2, illustrating a potential mechanism of SHP-1 to negatively regulate EPO signal transduction (Klingmuller et al. 1995). SHP-1 also has been shown to constitutively associate with Jak2 in EPO-dependent human leukemia cells, leading to the dephosphorylation of Jak2 through the N terminus of SHP-1 that is independent of the SH2 domain (Wu et al. 2000). SHP1 inhibit Jak2 can result in the inactivation of STATs (Pandey et al. 2009).

EPO and Wnt1

Wnt proteins are cysteine-rich glycosylated proteins that play important roles in stem cell development, vascular growth, the nervous system maturation, neurodegeneration, and cognition (Chong and Maiese 2004; Chong et al. 2010a; Maiese 2008). Wnt proteins have been categorized into two groups named canonical and noncanonical which function through different signaling pathways. Canonical Wnts include Wnt1, Wnt3a, and Wnt8 and function through β-catenin-dependent pathways. The noncanonical Wnts consist of Wnt4, Wnt5a, and Wnt11 and function through non-β-catenin-dependent pathways, such as the planar cell polarity pathway and the Wnt-calcium dependent pathway. Among these Wnts, Wnt1 is firstly identified as a proto-oncogene in mammary carcinomas through induction of mouse mammary tumor virus and also plays a critical role in neuronal development (Tang et al. 2002). Wnt1 can bind to the transmembrane receptor Frizzled and the co-receptor lipoprotein related protein 5 and 6 (LRP-5/6) followed by recruitment of disheveled, the cytoplasmic bridging molecule, to inhibit GSK-3β. The inhibition of GSK-3β prevents phosphorylation of β-catenin and its degradation.

The free β-catenin translocates to the nucleus where it activates lymphocyte enhancer factor (Lef) and T cell factor (Tcf)) leading to stimulation of Wnt1 response genes.

Interestingly, EPO can regulate Wnt1 to protect cells against apoptotic injury. In some scenarios, Wnt1 is necessary for EPO to preserve brain EC and microglial integrity, since administration of anti-Wnt1 neutralizing antibodies or gene silencing of Wnt1 block EPO protection during elevated glucose concentrations and Aβ exposure (Chong et al. 2007a; Shang et al. 2012). EPO promotes the phosphorylation of GSK-3β and translocation of β-catenin to the cell nucleus through Wnt1 and thereby to prevent apoptosis (Chong et al. 2011). EPO also promotes Wnt3a signaling in mesenchymal stem cells to protect against neurotoxicity (Danielyan et al. 2009). Wnt1 can regulate the expression of Apaf-1 and X-linked IAP for EPO to maintain microglial cell survival during OGD (Shang et al. 2011). In addition, EPO prevents against Aβ toxicity in microglia through Wnt1 mediated cell signaling pathways that involve modulation of PI3K, Bad, Bcl-x_L, and caspases (Shang et al. 2012).

EPO and Erythropoiesis

Circulating EPO binds to its receptor (EPOR) expressed on erythroid progenitor cells to promote erythropoiesis. Any impairment in the production of EPO will result in the deficiency of circulating erythrocytes and severe anemia. Recombinant human EPO also triggers the release of immature reticulocytes from the bone marrow into the circulation (Milarski and Saltiel 1994). Consequently, EPO has been widely used in the treatment of anemia during chronic renal failure and hematological malignancy (Chong et al. 2002b; Littlewood 2001). In patients with the anemia associated with end-stage renal disease, EPO can correct the anemia up to 97% patients, increasing the hematocrit levels by over 6 percentage, reducing the requirement of transfusion in patients who previously need red cell transfusions to maintain an adequate hematocrit, alleviating the symptoms of uremia including loss of energy and appetite (Krantz 1990). The dosage of EPO required to maintain a hematocrit level between 33% and 40% in patients on dialysis is intravenous (iv) injection of 225 U/kg/wk in 3 divided doses that is equal in effectiveness to a once-weekly iv administration of a dose of 429 U/kg/wk (Besarab 1993). Interestingly, the administration of EPO *via* the subcutaneous (sc) route is more efficient, reducing the required EPO dose by an average of 25% to 50% to achieve same level of hematocrit as iv administration (Besarab 1993). Moreover, the cost analysis indicates that the use of sc dosing two or three times weekly and total weekly dose of 120 U/kg is effective for the treatment of anemia in most patients on dialysis (Besarab 1993).

Several factors may influence the responsiveness to EPO. Due to the variable response to EPO, the broad range of EPO dose is required to maintain the targeted level of hematocrit, for example, 12.5 U/kg ~525 U/kg of iv EPO three times a week are needed to reach a hematocrit level of approximately 35% in hemodialysis patients with uncomplicated anemia (Eschbach et al. 1989). Analysis of the relationship between hematocrit and changes in the prescribed dose of EPO in cross annual national samples of hemodialysis patients from 1994 to 1998 indicates that male gender, older age, diabetes, higher hematocrit, and elevated weight, urea reduction ration, and transferrin saturation are associated with lower EPO requirement (Coladonato et al. 2002). Heavier patients are more sensitive to EPO than patients with less-than normal weight. It should be noted that low serum albumin has a strong association with higher EPO doses need and that men have significantly higher level of serum albumin and this may be the reason for men requiring less EPO. Older age and longer duration of dialysis tend to result in elevated hematocrit and less EPO requirement. In patients with end stage renal disease, EPO can induce normal hematocrit and the level can be maintained even after EPO application is stopped, implicating that native EPO secretion may be improved with time. The effectiveness of EPO in the treatment of anemia gives people an illustration that the higher hematocrit achieved with higher dose of EPO may be more beneficial to anemic patients. However, when hematocrit values rise above 40% in normal subjects, oxygen transport capacity decreases as a result of the decrease in cardiac index associated with a rise in blood viscosity. The optimal hematocrit for oxygen transport in patients with chronic renal disease should be lower than that in normal subjects because of decreased arterial and ventricular compliances and impaired cardiac index. Clinical trials have demonstrated that the higher target hemoglobin level (13.5 g/dl) with EPO in anemic patients of chronic kidney disease did not improve the quality of life compared with lower target hemoglobin (11.3 g/dl), but increased the risk of cardiovascular events (Singh et al. 2006). Similarly, both the target hemoglobin value of EPO treatment in the normal range (13.0 ~15.0 g /dl) and the subnormal range (10.5 ~11.5 g/dl) improve the general health and physical function in patients with chronic kidney disease, but higher incidence of hypertensive episodes and headache in the higher target hemoglobin group occurs (Drueke et al. 2006).

The analysis of the cost-effectiveness of EPO (epoetin alfa) therapy for anemia in patients with end-stage renal disease demonstrates that the cost including medication, laboratory, and transfusion costs for the six months increases by an average of $3000 on that time due to an increase in medication and laboratory costs even though the transfusion costs decreases (Moran et al. 1992).

EPO and Vascular Resistance

Increased vascular resistance and blood pressure can complicate recombinant human EPO during therapy for anemia. Several mechanisms have been proposed to account for the elevation in vascular resistance and the subsequent development of high blood pressure during EPO chronic administration.

Early studies attribute the increased blood viscosity as a result of elevated hemtocrit to high blood pressure during chronic treatment with EPO (Schaefer et al. 1988).

The application of EPO increases erythrocyte mass and blood viscosity (Steffen et al. 1989) and diminishes the hypoxic vasodilating response in uremic anemia (Roger et al. 1992).

Yet, further studies demonstrated that constant dosage and chronic administration of EPO in iron-deficient renal anemic patients did not increase blood pressure despite a dramatic increase in hematocrit by iron repletion (Kaupke et al. 1994). Thus, EPO can lead to hypertension during chronic treatment that appears to be independent of hematocrit levels.

The interaction between EPO and vasoactive substances may be a major contributor to the hypertensive effect of EPO. Treatment with EPO enhances vascular responsiveness to norepinephrine in renal failure (Hand et al. 1995) without an alteration of plasma catecholamine levels (Lebel et al. 1998). Further experiments that demonstrate an increase in intracellular calcium in vascular smooth muscle during EPO administration suggest that calcium mobilization also may contribute to the hypertension associated with recombinant human EPO treatment (Akimoto et al. 2000).

In addition, EPO may impair the balance between vasodilatory prostaglandin and vasoconstrictive components by reducing prostacyclin production and increasing the formation of prostaglandin $F_{2\alpha}$ and thromboxane B_2 (Bode-Boger et al. 1996).

EPO and Angiogenesis

Angiogenesis is the process of new capillary formation that extends the blood circulation from pre-existing vessels into an avascular area. This process involves vascular basal lamina formation, proliferation and migration of ECs, and alignment of migrating cells for tubular formation. Angiogenesis is physiologically active during embrogenesis (Risau 1997). In the adult, it occurs during more limited periods such as during menstruation and during some pathological conditions such as wound healing and tumor growth (Hanahan and Folkman 1996).

EPO can interact directly with ECs to elicit an angiogenic response. The proliferation and migration of ECs are crucial events in angiogenesis. Expression of the EPOR mRNA in ECs has been demonstrated in human umbilical veins (Anagnostou et al. 1994), bovine adrenal capillary (Anagnostou et al. 1990), and rat brain capillary (Yamaji et al. 1996). EPO can protect ECs against apoptotic cell death during oxidative stress (Chong et al. 2011; Chong et al. 2002a; Chong and Maiese 2007a). In cultured human and bovine ECs, EPO not only stimulates proliferation, but also enhances the migration of ECs (Anagnostou et al. 1990). Other investigations illustrate the migration of ECs on the Matrigel surface to form branching and anastomosing tubes in response to EPO exposure (Ribatti et al. 1999). In addition, angiogenesis has been observed in rat aortic rings four days following incubation with EPO in reconstituted basement membrane matrix (Carlini et al. 1995). Application of EPO prior to cerebral ischemia enhances the expression of EPOR on ECs in the penumbra region several days (3-24 days) after ischemia. EPO induces an increase in the expression of angiogenic factors Tie-2, angiopoietin-2, and vascular endothelial growth factor (VEGF) and the proliferation of ECs, resulting in an increase of regional cerebral blood flow, suggesting that EPO upregulates the EPOR level in vascular ECs and enhances angiogenesis (Li et al. 2007).

Current work has illustrated that EPO can promote intussusceptive microvascular growth in the heart, suggesting that the protective effect of EPO on ischemic heart disease may be a partial result from an increase in myocardium blood supply as a result of the generation of new blood vessels (Crivellato et al. 2004). EPO can prevent serum-free medium induced apoptosis and VEGF release in marrow stromal cells (MSC). Combined the transplantation of MSCs with EPO into the ischemic heart significantly reduces cardiac infarct size, improves cardiac function, and increases the capillary density suggesting that EPO promotes the angiogenic effect of MSCs (Zhang et al. 2007). Further study suggest that EPO can promotes the migration capacity of bone marrow derived cells into ischemic tissue to improve angiogenesis and perfusion (Brunner et al. 2012). Given that endothelial progenitor cell (EPC) participate in vascular repair and angiogenesis through its differentiation into ECs, EPC transplantation into ischemic myocardium has been performed to improve cardiac function.

Application of EPO during MI in mice promotes the survival of EPCs transplanted into peri-infarct myocardium and enhances autologue EPC mobilization, resulting in an increase in microvessel density, inhibition of apoptosis, and prevention of fibrosis in the peri-infarct myocardium (Cheng et al. 2012).

EPO and Coronary Heart Disease

The cytoporotectve effects of EPO both *in vitro* and *in vivo* have been demonstrated during cardiac ischemia and reperfusion injury. In isolated hearts subjected to ischemia-reperfusion, treatment with EPO twenty-four hours following injury can reduce apoptosis in cardiomyocytes, limit myocardial infarct size, and promote functional recovery of the heart (Cai et al. 2003). Parenteral administration of EPO also is sufficient to induce dramatic protection against ischemia-reperfusion injury in the heart (Semenza 2004). A more recent study has demonstrated that EPO treatment either prior to or during myocardial ischemia/reperfusion can protect against myocardial cell apoptosis and decrease infarct size, resulting in an enhanced cardiac function and recovery, including left ventricular contractility (Parsa et al. 2004). In the isolated rat heart following ischemia/reperfusion experiments, beneficial effects of treatment with EPO also have been shown to reduce cellular necrosis and improve post-ischemic recovery of left ventricular pressure significantly (van der Meer et al. 2004; Wright et al. 2004).

At the onset of coronary artery occlusion, EPO administered can significantly inhibit apoptosis in the central region of myocardial ischemia (Tramontano et al. 2003). Even in acute scenarios following coronary artery ligation, EPO leads to a decrease in apoptotic cells by fifty percent in the myocardium and significantly improves cardiac function (Moon et al. 2003; Parsa et al. 2003). Single dose intramyocardial EPO (3000 IU/kg) administration can promote early intracardiac cell proliferation, which may at least in part contribute to myocardial functional improvement (Gabel et al. 2009).

Intracardiac EPO injection also enhances the expression of stromal cell derived factor-1 (SDF-1) and stem cell proliferation to beneficially restore myocardial functions following MI (Gabel et al. 2009).

In acute phase of myocardial infarction (MI), the plasma level of EPO is significantly increased, implicating and initiating the further investigation of the role of EPO in MI (Anton Martinez et al. 1997). Further study demonstrated that a high serum EPO level correlated to a smaller infarct size in patients with acute MI subjected to successful primary PCI (Namiuchi et al. 2005).

A single intraperitoneal injection of recombinant human EPO (3,000 IU/kg) immediately after the coronary artery ligation reduces apoptosis in the myocardial area at risk by 50% 24 h later and reduces the infarct size to 15-25% of control animals 8 weeks after ischemia (Moon et al. 2003). Although delayed administration of EPO fails to reduce the infarct volume, EPO given 3 weeks after MI can improve cardiac function with 34% reduction in left ventricular end-diastolic pressure and 46% decrease in atrial natriuretic peptide level accompanied by increased capillary density, elevated capillary-to-myocyte ratio, and a partial reversal of beta- myosin heavy chain (van der Meer et al. 2005).

The efficacy of EPO in experimental MI has time window and dose association. For example, a single intravenous injection of EPO immediately following MI in a dose of 150 IU/kg was as effective as 3,000 IU/kg in apoptosis reduction 24 hrs late, the reduction of infarct size measured 4 weeks following ischemia, attenuation of progressive left ventricle dilatation, and ejection fraction improvement. The efficacy of 3000 IU/kg EPO can be extended to delayed administration to 12 hrs following ischemia. The 150 IU/kg EPO dose was effective only within 4 h post-MI. The results suggest that higher doses EPO extend the therapeutic window to a longer period of time (Moon et al. 2005). Yet, multiple dosing of EPO (3000 IU/kg) after myocardial infarction in rats did not show added therapeutic benefits over those achieved by a single dose (Moon et al. 2006). In a dog model of permanent ligation of the coronary artery, intravenously administered EPO (1,000 IU/kg) immediately, 6 hr, or 1 week after the ligation and the results indicate that closest administration of EPO to the onset of ischemia results the best efficacy, including regional blood flow and cardiac function improvement (Hirata et al. 2006). In a pig model of a 90-minute balloon occlusion of the left anterior descending coronary artery, prolonged EPO therapy is safe and leads to an increase in viable myocardium, increased vascular density, and improved left ventricular function (Angeli et al. 2010).

However, treatment with high dose of EPO (5000 IU/kg/day) the day before surgery, the day of, then for 5 days in rats underwent coronary artery occlusion, there is no improvement in left ventricle remodeling and cardiac function 6 weeks later (Hale et al. 2005). Even single high dose (5000 IU/kg) can reduce left ventricle function and aggravate the remodeling following MI, repeated low dose of EPO (750 IU/kg/week) improves the left ventricle function (Ben-Dor et al. 2007). As a result, to achieve the beneficial effect of EPO during MI, close controlled dosage of EPO is critical in the treatment of MI.

In addition to the correction of anemia, the beneficial effects of EPO on heart failure result from a direct protection of the myocardial cells. As a result, EPO is considered to be appropriate for the treatment of patients with heart failure following anemia or anemia accompanying heart failure. Early studies have indicated that administration of EPO can lead to a decrease in left ventricular hypertrophy, inhibit left ventricular dilatation, and increase left ventricular ejection fraction, stroke volume, and cardiac output, suggesting cardiac function improvement in patients with congestive heart failure resulted from anemia correction (Goldberg et al. 1992; Low-Friedrich et al. 1991). Other *in vivo* studies have illustrated that treatment with EPO can increase cardiac cell proliferation in neonatal rats, reduce myocardiocyte apoptosis during ischemia-reperfusion injury, and improve left ventricular function (Calvillo et al. 2003; Moon et al. 2003; Parsa et al. 2003).

In patients with acute MI treated with aspirin and clopidogrel, recombinant human EPO (200 U/kg iv daily for 3 consecutive days) did not alter bleeding time, platelet function, von Willebrand factor levels, soluble P-selectin, or soluble Fas ligand levels, but significantly increased expression of EPOR, VEGF, receptor Flt-1, and phosphorylated PI3K in peripheral blood mononuclear cells (Tang et al. 2009). Short-term high-dose EPO (33000 IU, before PCI, 24, and 48 after) administration in patients with acute MI treated by PCI and standard anti-platelet therapy decreases infarct size and increases the levels of circulating CD34+ cells, increases the expression of anti-apoptotic, pro-angiogenic and anti-inflammatory genes, such as Akt, NF-κB, VEGF receptor-2, and the EPORs, and decreases the expression of the pro-apoptotic caspase-3, TP53, and pro-inflammatory IL12a (Ferrario et al. 2011). The clinical relevance of these results needs to be confirmed in specifically tailored trials. These data suggest that EPO is safe at a low dosage in acute MI.

Randomized control studies in patients with mild anemia and severe or resistant congestive heart failure have demonstrated that EPO in combination with intravenous iron can lead to increased left ventricular ejection fraction and a reduction in hospitalization days by almost eighty percent (Silverberg et al. 2001). Additional investigations involving subcutaneous EPO in diabetics and non-diabetics with severe, resistant congestive heart failure has been shown to decrease breathlessness and/or fatigue, increase left ventricular ejection fraction, and significantly decrease the number of hospitalization days (Silverberg et al. 2003). In patients with moderate to severe chronic heart failure, the peak oxygen consumption and exercise duration of patients are significantly increased following treatment with EPO, suggesting that EPO can enhance exercise capacity in patients with heart failure. As a result, work has supported the premise that EPO can function as a novel cytoprotectant against acute or chronic ischemic heart disease by enhancing cardiac cell survival and proliferation, increasing cardiovascular blood flow, and improving heart remodeling and function.

However, a single intravenous bolus of EPO in patients who had successfully reperfusion with percutaneous coronary intervention (PCI) 4 hours ago did not reduce infarct volume, but may have tendency to increase the infarct volume in older patients (Najjar et al. 2011). Systemic review and meta-analysis of randomized controlled 13 trials of EPO indicate that EPO therapy did not improve ejection fraction, had no effect on infarct size, did not decrease the risk of total adverse cardiac events, failed to decrease the risk of heart failure, had no effect on the risk of stent thrombosis, suggesting that in some scenarios, there is no beneficial effect of EPO application in acute MI (Gao et al. 2012) and the role of EPO in MI need to be further elucidation.

Cellular Protection of EPO in the CNS

EPO has been demonstrated to robustly protect cells in the CNS against a variety of insults. As a hematopoietic growth factor, EPO is fascinating to enhance the survival of a number of cells in the CNS including neurons, glial cells, and brain ECs {Lykissas, 2007 #8362; Maiese, 2004 #6148; Maiese, 2005 #6261; Kato, 2011 #3287; Yoo, 2009 #3557; Chong, 2007 #3035; Chong, 2002 #1948}. Treatment with EPO in the cultures of human neuroblastoma (SH-SY5Y) cells prevents staurosporine, tumor necrosis factor (TNF)-alpha, or hypoxia induced apoptosis (Wenker et al. 2010) and preserves cell integrity during oxygen glucose deprivation (OGD) (Chong et al. 2012b). Early application of EPO protects against hypoxia-induced retinal neuronal apoptosis, although delayed use of EPO may otherwise enhance pathological neovascularization in retina (Chen et al. 2008).

In primary cultures, EPO is strongly expressed in astrocytes, whereas EPOR is only detected in neurons. Interestingly, neurons in mixed neuronal/astrocytic are injured at significantly reduced level than in neuron-rich cultures after hypoxia (Liu et al. 1999). Application of recombinant human EPO (0.1 U/ml) within 6 h before or after hypoxia significantly increased neuronal survival in both neuronal and neuronal/astrocytic cultures, suggesting that both intrinsic and extrinsic EPO can protect neurons against hypoxia/ischemia (Liu et al. 2006). Similarly, EPO also can protect microglia and cerebral ECs against anoxia (Chong et al. 2002a) and OGD (Chong et al. 2007b; Chong and Maiese 2007a; Shang et al. 2011).

In addition, EPO can preserve the integrity of cerebral ECs and reduce EC apoptosis during elevated glucose concentrations (Chong et al. 2011; Chong et al. 2007c; Hou et al. 2011).

Endogenous EPO produced in astrocytes under hypoxic condition can protect oligodendrocyte precursor cells against hypoxia/reoxygenation injury, since gene silence of EPO in astrocytes and EPOR in oligodendrocytes result in an increased cell injury during hypoxic stress (Kato et al. 2011).

In particular, EPO also exhibits strong protection during neurotoxicity. In primary cultured hippocampal neurons, free radical exposure with nitric oxide (NO) donors induces both genomic DNA fragmentation and phosphatidylserine exposure; in contrast, application of EPO at the concentrations from 0.01 to 10 U/ml significantly reduces apoptotic cell injury; the protection was abolished by co-application of EPO neutralizing antibody that can bind to EPO and block the biological activity of EPO (Chong et al. 2003b). Administration of EPO also represents a viable option for the prevention of retinal cell and hippocampal neuronal apoptosis during glutamate toxicity (Morishita et al. 1997; Zhong et al. 2007). L-3,4-dihydroxyphenylalanine (L-DOPA) induced oxidative stress and apoptotic injury in PC12 cells can also be prevented by EPO treatment (Park et al. 2011; Wu et al. 2007), suggesting its potential in the therapy of Parkinson's disease (PD). The amyloid-beta (Aβ) exposure induces apoptotic injury in hippocampal neurons, microglia, and PC12 cells; administration of EPO can robustly inhibit apoptosis and improve cell survival (Chong et al. 2005b; Ma et al. 2009; Shang et al. 2012).

There exists a therapeutic window and a temporal pattern of EPO for cytoprotection. Neuroprotection with EPO has been achieved in a limited concentration range, for example, EPO at the concentration between 0.1 and 50 U/ml significantly promotes neuronal survival against Aβ (Chong et al. 2005a), or at the range from 0.01 to 10 U/ml against NO toxicity (Chong et al. 2003b).

No significant efficacy of EPO has been observed at the concentrations less than 0.01 U/ml or greater than 50 U/ml (Chong et al. 2003b). The protection of EPO has also been associated with the temporal scenario of EPO application. Administration of EPO to hippocampal neuron cultures up to six hours following NO exposure can offer significant protection. Yet, treatment with EPO that is delayed as long as twelve hours post NO exposure doses not increase the neuronal survival, suggesting that EPO may require sufficient time to induce its protective cascade prior to the occurrence of irreversible stage of cell injury.

Yet, prolonged incubation of EPO reduces the capacity of EPO to offer neuroprotection, the greatest protection has been achieved with EPO administered at the time closest to the onset of injury (Chong et al. 2003b). The possible mechanism underlying the concentration and temporal pattern of EPO protection may associate with the formation of anti-EPO antibody and down-regulation of EPOR following prolonged exposure to EPO (Casadevall et al. 2002; Verdier et al. 2000).

EPO can stimulate neuronal stem cells (NSCs) to promote the number of neuronal progenitors (Maiese et al. 2004; Shingo et al. 2001). EPO infusion into the adult lateral ventricles increases newly generated cells migrating to the olfactory bulb and increases new olfactory bulb interneurons accompanied by a decrease in the numbers of NSCs in the subventricular zone (SVZ) (Shingo et al. 2001).

Given that neural progenitor cells expressing a higher level of EPOR, EPO can promote the proliferation of embryonic neural progenitor cells. In contrast, embryonic brain in EPOR null mice exhibits increased neural cell apoptosis and impaired neural cell proliferation in the adult hippocampus and SVZ (Chen et al. 2007).

During neonatal stroke, EPO application can increase the percentage of newly generated neurons, decrease newly generated astrocytes (Gonzalez et al. 2007), and increase both neurogenesis in the SVZ and migration of neuronal progenitors into the ischemic cortex and striatum (Wang et al. 2004).

In adult rats, EPO also increases the proliferation and differentiation of neural progenitor cells and neurite outgrowth in SVZ (Wang et al. 2006), suggesting the neuroregenerative activity of EPO and its potential roles in neurodegenerative diseases (Byts and Siren 2009).

EPO and Neurodegenerative Diseases

EPO and Alzheimer's Disease

Alzheimer's disease (AD) is characterized by two pathologic hallmarks that consist of extracellular plaques of Aβ peptide aggregates and intracellular neurofibrillary tangles composed of hyperphosphorylated microtubular protein tau and lead to a progressive deterioration of cognitive function with loss of memory (Chong et al. 2005d). Application of EPO or its non-erythropoietic carbamylated derivative (CEPO) to mouse has been demonstrated to not only improve spatial and non-spatial recognition memory and also promote neurogenesis in the dentate gyrus of the hippocampus (Leconte et al. 2011). Intraperitoneal injection of EPO improves sensorimotor function in mice during neonatal hypoxia, and prevents striatum atrophy, hippocampus injury, and white matter loss (Fan et al. 2011). In aged (Tg2576) mice, in which EPOR expresses in the cortex and hippocampus, EPO improves contextual memory and decreases the amount of amyloid plaque and Aβ (Lee et al. 2012). An interesting investigation indicates that human mesenchymal stem cells (hMSCs) exposed to EPO demonstrates a cholinergic neuron-like phenotype with an increase in cellular choline acetyltransferase, acetylcholine (Ach) and Ach receptor, suggesting that EPO promotes the differentiation of MSCs into cholinergic neurons (Danielyan et al. 2009). Moreover, EPO can accelerate the degradation of Aβ in MSCs *via* increasing neprilysin (Danielyan et al. 2009). In addition, EPO has been shown to prevent Aβ induced tau hyperphosphorylation in SH-SY5Y cells *via* a mechanism that is dependent on the PI3K/Akt-GSK-3β signaling pathway (Sun et al. 2008). These improving effects of EPO on experimental AD suggest its possible therapeutic role in the management of AD.

EPO and Parkinson's Disease

Parkinson disease (PD) is a movement disorder characterized by resting tremor, rigidity and bradykinesia. The pathophysiological basis of the symptoms rests upon the degeneration of dopaminergic neurons (DA) in the substantia nigra (SN). EPO appears to robustly prevent 1-3, 4-dihydroxyphenylalanine toxicity through reducing caspase 3 activation (Park et al. 2011) and represses the expression of the pro-apoptotic protein p53 up-regulated modulator of apoptosis (PUMA) in the 1-methyl-4-phenylpyridinium (MPP^+) model of PD in rats (Kook et al. 2011). In a rat model of PD with intrastriatal 6-hydroxydopamine (6-OHDA) injection, EPO reduces behavioral impairment, prevents the loss of DA, promotes neurogenesis in the SVZ, and inhibits apoptotic injury of neurons through activating Akt (Kadota et al. 2009; Signore et al. 2006). EPO (1-3 U/ml) can protect both dopaminergic cell line (MN9D) and primary DA against 6-OHDA induced apoptosis through activating PI3K/Akt (Signore et al. 2006). When EPO is administered with transplantation of embryonic ventral mesencephalic DA neurons into the striatum, EPO can improve the survival of grafted neurons and significantly increase functional improvements (Kanaan et al. 2006). Intrastriatal but not systemic administration of EPO can reduce microglia activation in SN, protect nigral DA against 6-OHDA, and improve neurobehavioral outcome in a rats (Xue et al. 2007). In addition, adeno-associated viral serotype 9 (AAV9) vector mediated deliver of the human EPO gene into the brain of 6-OHDA-lesioned rats robustly promotes the expression of the human EPO gene in the striatum and the SN, prevents DA neuronal loss, attenuates the rotational and spontaneous forelimb use asymmetry (Xue et al. 2010).

EPO and Epilepsy

Although EPO was found to induce seizure in patients with dialysis, it has been considered as the result of hypertension and thrombosis (Zhu and Perazella 2006). More recent works have demonstrated that EPO exert favorable action for epilepsy. Administration of the single dose of EPO (1000 U/kg, ip) after an acute hypoxia in postnatal rats increases the latency to forelimb clonus seizures, reduces seizure duration, and reduces the neuronal loss in hippocampus (Mikati et al. 2007). In an adult animal model of seizure induced by kainic acid in Fischer 344 rats, continuous intraventricular infusion of EPO significantly reduces mortality rate, seizure severity, apoptotic cell death, and abnormal cell proliferation in the hippocampus, in contrast, anti-EPO antibody in non-EPO-treated animals worsens seizures and CA1 neuronal cell death, suggesting that both endogenous and exogenous EPO are effective to attenuate seizure induced by neurotoxicity through blockade of epileptogenic cell formation (Kondo et al. 2009). EPO also can prevent spontaneous seizure following febrile seizure and this may be associated with regulatory efficacy of EPO on the early inflammatory responses and the molecular alterations after febrile seizures (Jung et al. 2011).

Intraperitoneal injection of EPO (10 U/g) 40 min after lithium-pilocarpine injection in neonatal rats, which induces status epilepticus, can prevent status epilepticus induced neuronal cell death and apoptosis in dentate gyrus of hippocampus (Sozmen et al. 2012).

EPO and Multiple Sclerosis

Multiple sclerosis (MS) is a heterogeneous inflammatory demyelinating disease of the CNS and the most common cause of neurological disability in young adults. EPO has been demonstrated to improve the outcomes in experimental MS through its neuroprotective and neuroregenerative capability (Bartels et al. 2008). In experimental autoimmune encephalomyelitis (EAE), the most common used model of MS, intraperitoneal administration of EPO at doses of 500-5000 U/kg daily for 12-13 days after immunization with myelin basic protein (MBP), delays the onset of EAE, reduces inflammation, and decreases its clinical score (Agnello et al. 2002). Delayed administration of EPO and its non-erythropoietic derivatives CEPO and asialo-EPO also decreases the EAE-associated production of inflammatory cytokines including TNF-α, IL-1β and IL-1Ra, in the spinal cord, and IFN-γ by peripheral lymphocytes, in a mouse model of chronic murine EAE induced by immunization with the myelin oligodendrocyte glycoprotein peptide, suggesting that EPO provide a novel avenue to prevent the progression of MS through its anti-neuroinflammatory action (Savino et al. 2006). In addition, EPO can also promote the proliferation of oligodendrocyte progenitor cells and improve neurological function in EAE (Zhang et al. 2005). Further study indicates that EPO ameliorates neurological symptoms in mice with cuprizone induction of demyelination may through reducing inflammation associated axonal degeneration in white matter tracts (Hagemeyer et al. 2012). In addition, EPO can promote oligodendrogenesis and enhance the remyelination that may link to increased EPOR expression in spinal cord slice culture after lysolecithin-induced demyelination (Cho et al. 2012).

EPO and Motor Neuron Diseases

Amyotrophic lateral sclerosis (ALS) is the most common motor neuron diseases characterized by rapidly progressive weakness, muscle atrophy, and fasciculations.

The progressive decline of EPO in the cerebrospinal fluid has been observed in patients with ALS (Janik et al. 2010), suggesting the ability of EPO to antagonize the progression of ALS. EPO can protect motor neurons against glutamate-induced apoptosis (Naganska et al. 2010).

In a mouse model of ALS, EPO delays the onset of motor deterioration in transgenic superoxide dismutase G93A female mice but without prolonging their survival (Grunfeld et al. 2007), reduces the loss of motor neurons, and prevents inflammatory reaction (Koh et al. 2007)].

Conclusion

EPO is produced and EPO receptor is expressed throughout the body. The biological activities of EPO is multiple by governing a series of cell signal transduction pathways that involve Jak2, PI3K/Akt, STATs, ERK, FoxO3a, GSK-3β, NF-κB, mTOR, and Wnt1.

Although a variety of cell signaling pathways have been identified to regulate the cytoprotection of EPO, the new targets of EPO and their interactions for cytoprotection is still accumulating. Given the biological function of EPO in the cardiovascular and nervous systems, EPO has been considered as a potential candidate for coronary heart diseases and neurodegenerative diseases, but to realize the goal of practically use of EPO in these system diseases has a long way to go.

In addition, due to its erythropoietic and vascular effects, chronic use of EPO can increase red blood cells, blood viscosity, and blood vessel resistance to increase the incidence of thromboembolic complications and lead to hypertension, limiting its chronic use.

In some cases, higher doses may be required for EPO to protect cells than to stimulate red blood cell production (Velly et al. 2010). To achieve its cytoprotective effects in the CNS, the systemic administration of high dose EPO raises more concerns about its complications in the vascular system. To avert this erythropoietic effects of EPO when it is applied for cytoprotection, some non-erythropoietic derivatives of EPO with cytoprotective activity have been developed, including carbamylated EPO (CEPO) (Leist et al. 2004) and asialo-EPO (Erbayraktar et al. 2003), facilitating chronic use of EPO. The non-erythropoietic EPO development may hold a promise for its application in diseases other than anemia.

References

Agnello, D., Bigini, P., Villa, P., Mennini, T., Cerami, A., Brines, M. L., Ghezzi, P. (2002) Erythropoietin exerts an anti-inflammatory effect on the

CNS in a model of experimental autoimmune encephalomyelitis. *Brain Res.* 952:128-134

Akimoto, T., Kusano, E., Inaba, T., Iimura, O., Takahashi, H., Ikeda, H., Ito, C., Ando, Y., Ozawa, K., Asano, Y. (2000) Erythropoietin regulates vascular smooth muscle cell apoptosis by a phosphatidylinositol 3 kinase-dependent pathway. *Kidney Int.* 58:269-282

Anagnostou, A., Lee, E. S., Kessimian, N., Levinson, R., Steiner, M. (1990) Erythropoietin has a mitogenic and positive chemotactic effect on endothelial cells. *Proc. Natl. Acad. Sci. US* 87:5978-5982

Anagnostou, A., Liu, Z., Steiner, M., Chin, K., Lee, E. S., Kessimian, N., Noguchi, C. T. (1994) Erythropoietin receptor mRNA expression in human endothelial cells. *Proc. Natl. Acad. Sci. US* 91:3974-3978

Angeli, F. S., Amabile, N., Burjonroppa, S., Shapiro, M., Bartlett, L., Zhang, Y., Virmani, R., Chatterjee, K., Boyle, A., Grossman, W., Yeghiazarians, Y. (2010) Prolonged therapy with erythropoietin is safe and prevents deterioration of left ventricular systolic function in a porcine model of myocardial infarction. *J. Card. Fail.* 16:579-589

Anton Martinez, J., Ojeda Ortego, J., Gonzalez Blanco, P., Gutierrez Sampedro, N., Palma Nieto, J. C., Leon Garcia, L. A. (1997) [Increased levels of erythropoietin in the initial phase of acute myocardial infarction]. *An. Med. Interna.* 14:459-461

Bachmann, E., Weber, E. (1993) Recirculating, retrograde heart perfusion according to the Langendorff method for evaluation of MTG--methyl-2-tetradecylglycidate, McNeil 3716--cardiomyopathy. *Pharmacol. Toxicol.* 72:98-106

Bartels, C., Spate, K., Krampe, H., Ehrenreich, H. (2008) Recombinant Human Erythropoietin: Novel Strategies for Neuroprotective/Neuro-regenerative Treatment of Multiple Sclerosis. *Ther. Adv. Neurol. Disord.* 1:193-206

Ben-Dor, I., Hardy, B., Fuchs, S., Kaganovsky, E., Kadmon, E., Sagie, A., Coleman, R., Mansur, M., Politi, B., Fraser, A., Harell, D., Okon, E., Battler, A., Haim, M. (2007) Repeated low-dose of erythropoietin is associated with improved left ventricular function in rat acute myocardial infarction model. *Cardiovasc. Drugs Ther.* 21:339-346

Bernaudin, M., Bellail, A., Marti, H. H., Yvon, A., Vivien, D., Duchatelle, I., Mackenzie, E. T., Petit, E. (2000) Neurons and astrocytes express EPO mRNA: oxygen-sensing mechanisms that involve the redox-state of the brain. *Glia* 30:271-278.

Besarab, A. (1993) Optimizing epoetin therapy in end-stage renal disease: the case for subcutaneous administration. *Am. J. Kidney Dis.* 22:13-22

Bode-Boger, S. M., Boger, R. H., Kuhn, M., Radermacher, J., Frolich, J. C. (1996) Recombinant human erythropoietin enhances vasoconstrictor tone via endothelin-1 and constrictor prostanoids. *Kidney Int.* 50:1255-1261

Bonsdorff, E., Jalavisto, E. (1948) A humoral mechanism in anoxic erythrocytosis. *Acta. Physiol. Scand.* 16:150-170

Brockmoller, J., Kochling, J., Weber, W., Looby, M., Roots, I., Neumayer, H. H. (1992) The pharmacokinetics and pharmacodynamics of recombinant human erythropoietin in haemodialysis patients. *Br. J. Clin. Pharmacol.* 34:499-508

Brunet, A., Bonni, A., Zigmond, M. J., Lin, M. Z., Juo, P., Hu, L. S., Anderson, M. J., Arden, K. C., Blenis, J., Greenberg, M. E. (1999) Akt promotes cell survival by phosphorylating and inhibiting a Forkhead transcription factor. *Cell* 96:857-868

Brunner, S., Huber, B. C., Weinberger, T., Vallaster, M., Wollenweber, T., Gerbitz, A., Hacker, M., Franz, W. M. (2012) Migration of bone marrow-derived cells and improved perfusion after treatment with erythropoietin in a murine model of myocardial infarction. *J. Cell Mol. Med.* 16:152-159

Bunn, H. F., Gu, J., Huang, L. E., Park, J. W., Zhu, H. (1998) Erythropoietin: a model system for studying oxygen-dependent gene regulation. *J. Exp. Biol.* 201 (Pt 8):1197-1201

Byts, N., Siren, A. L. (2009) Erythropoietin: a multimodal neuroprotective agent. *Exp. Transl. Stroke Med.* 1:4

Cai, Z., Manalo, D. J., Wei, G., Rodriguez, E. R., Fox-Talbot, K., Lu, H., Zweier, J. L., Semenza, G. L. (2003) Hearts from rodents exposed to intermittent hypoxia or erythropoietin are protected against ischemia-reperfusion injury. *Circulation* 108:79-85

Calvillo, L., Latini, R., Kajstura, J., Leri, A., Anversa, P., Ghezzi, P., Salio, M., Cerami, A., Brines, M. (2003) Recombinant human erythropoietin protects the myocardium from ischemia-reperfusion injury and promotes beneficial remodeling. *Proc. Natl. Acad. Sci. US* 100:4802-4806

Carlini, R. G., Reyes, A. A., Rothstein, M. (1995) Recombinant human erythropoietin stimulates angiogenesis in vitro. *Kidney Int.* 47:740-745

Carnot, P., DeFlandre, C. (1906) Sur l" active hematopoietique de serum au cours de la regeneration di sang. *CR Acad. Sci.* 143:384-386

Casadevall, N., Nataf, J., Viron, B., Kolta, A., Kiladjian, J. J., Martin-Dupont, P., Michaud, P., Papo, T., Ugo, V., Teyssandier, I., Varet, B., Mayeux, P.

(2002) Pure red-cell aplasia and antierythropoietin antibodies in patients treated with recombinant erythropoietin. *N Engl. J. Med.* 346:469-475

Chavez, J. C., Agani, F., Pichiule, P., LaManna, J. C. (2000) Expression of hypoxia-inducible factor-1alpha in the brain of rats during chronic hypoxia. *J. Appl. Physiol.* 89:1937-1942

Chavez, J. C., Baranova, O., Lin, J., Pichiule, P. (2006) The transcriptional activator hypoxia inducible factor 2 (HIF-2/EPAS-1) regulates the oxygen-dependent expression of erythropoietin in cortical astrocytes. *J. Neurosci.* 26:9471-9481

Chen, J., Connor, K. M., Aderman, C. M., Smith, L. E. (2008) Erythropoietin deficiency decreases vascular stability in mice. *J. Clin. Invest.* 118:526-533

Chen, L., Xu, B., Liu, L., Luo, Y., Yin, J., Zhou, H., Chen, W., Shen, T., Han, X., Huang, S. (2010) Hydrogen peroxide inhibits mTOR signaling by activation of AMPKalpha leading to apoptosis of neuronal cells. *Lab. Invest.* 90:762-773

Chen, Z. Y., Asavaritikrai, P., Prchal, J. T., Noguchi, C. T. (2007) Endogenous erythropoietin signaling is required for normal neural progenitor cell proliferation. *J. Biol. Chem.* 282:25875-25883

Cheng, Y., Hu, R., Lv, L., Ling, L., Jiang, S. (2012) Erythropoietin improves the efficiency of endothelial progenitor cell therapy after myocardial infarction in mice: effects on transplanted cell survival and autologous endothelial progenitor cell mobilization. *J. Surg. Res.* 176:e47-55

Chikuma, M., Masuda, S., Kobayashi, T., Nagao, M., Sasaki, R. (2000) Tissue-specific regulation of erythropoietin production in the murine kidney, brain, and uterus. *Am. J. Physiol. Endocrinol. Metab.* 279:E1242-1248

Cho, Y. K., Kim, G., Park, S., Sim, J. H., Won, Y. J., Hwang, C. H., Yoo, J. Y., Hong, H. N. (2012) Erythropoietin promotes oligodendrogenesis and myelin repair following lysolecithin-induced injury in spinal cord slice culture. *Biochem. Biophys. Res. Commun.* 417:753-759

Chong, Z. Z., Hou, J., Shang, Y. C., Wang, S., Maiese, K. (2011) EPO relies upon novel signaling of Wnt1 that requires Akt1, FoxO3a, GSK-3beta, and beta-catenin to foster vascular integrity during experimental diabetes. *Curr. Neurovasc. Res.* 8:103-120

Chong, Z. Z., Kang, J., Li, F., Maiese, K. (2005a) mGluRI targets microglial activation and selectively prevents neuronal cell engulfment through Akt and caspase dependent pathways. *Curr. Neurovasc. Res.* 2:197-211

Chong, Z. Z., Kang, J. Q., Maiese, K. (2002a) Erythropoietin is a novel vascular protectant through activation of Akt1 and mitochondrial modulation of cysteine proteases. *Circulation* 106:2973-2979

Chong, Z. Z., Kang, J. Q., Maiese, K. (2002b) Hematopoietic factor erythropoietin fosters neuroprotection through novel signal transduction cascades. *J. Cereb. Blood Flow Metab.* 22:503-514

Chong, Z. Z., Kang, J. Q., Maiese, K. (2003a) Apaf-1, Bcl-xL, cytochrome c, and caspase-9 form the critical elements for cerebral vascular protection by erythropoietin. *J. Cereb. Blood Flow Metab.* 23:320-330

Chong, Z. Z., Kang, J. Q., Maiese, K. (2003b) Erythropoietin fosters both intrinsic and extrinsic neuronal protection through modulation of microglia, Akt1, Bad, and caspase-mediated pathways. *Br. J. Pharmacol.* 138:1107-1118

Chong, Z. Z., Kang, J. Q., Maiese, K. (2004) AKT1 drives endothelial cell membrane asymmetry and microglial activation through Bcl-xL and caspase 1, 3, and 9. *Exp. Cell Res.* 296:196-207

Chong, Z. Z., Li, F., Maiese, K. (2005b) Activating Akt and the brain's resources to drive cellular survival and prevent inflammatory injury. *Histol. Histopathol.* 20:299-315

Chong, Z. Z., Li, F., Maiese, K. (2005c) Erythropoietin requires NF-kappaB and its nuclear translocation to prevent early and late apoptotic neuronal injury during beta-amyloid toxicity. *Curr. Neurovasc. Res.* 2:387-399

Chong, Z. Z., Li, F., Maiese, K. (2005d) Stress in the brain: novel cellular mechanisms of injury linked to Alzheimer's disease. *Brain Res. Brain Res. Rev.* 49:1-21

Chong, Z. Z., Li, F., Maiese, K. (2006) Group I metabotropic receptor neuroprotection requires Akt and its substrates that govern FOXO3a, Bim, and beta-catenin during oxidative stress. *Curr. Neurovasc. Res.* 3:107-117

Chong, Z. Z., Li, F., Maiese, K. (2007a) Cellular demise and inflammatory microglial activation during beta-amyloid toxicity are governed by Wnt1 and canonical signaling pathways. *Cell Signal* 19:1150-1162

Chong, Z. Z., Li, F., Maiese, K. (2007b) The pro-survival pathways of mTOR and protein kinase B target glycogen synthase kinase-3beta and nuclear factor-kappaB to foster endogenous microglial cell protection. *Int. J. Mol. Med.* 19:263-272

Chong, Z. Z., Maiese, K. (2004) Targeting WNT, protein kinase B, and mitochondrial membrane integrity to foster cellular survival in the nervous system. *Histol. Histopathol.* 19:495-504

Chong, Z. Z., Maiese, K. (2007a) Erythropoietin involves the phosphatedylinositol 3-kinase pathway, 14-3-3 protein and FOXO3a nuclear trafficking to preserve endothelial cell integrity. *Br. J. Pharmacol.* 150: 839-850

Chong, Z. Z., Maiese, K. (2007b) The Src homology 2 domain tyrosine phosphatases SHP-1 and SHP-2: diversified control of cell growth, inflammation, and injury. *Histol. Histopathol.* 22:1251-1267

Chong, Z. Z., Shang, Y. C., Hou, J., Maiese, K. (2010a) Wnt1 neuroprotection translates into improved neurological function during oxidant stress and cerebral ischemia through AKT1 and mitochondrial apoptotic pathways. *Oxid. Med. Cell Longev.* 3:153-165

Chong, Z. Z., Shang, Y. C., Maiese, K. (2007c) Vascular injury during elevated glucose can be mitigated by erythropoietin and Wnt signaling. *Curr. Neurovasc. Res.* 4:194-204

Chong, Z. Z., Shang, Y. C., Wang, S., Maiese, K. (2012a) A Critical Kinase Cascade in Neurological Disorders: PI 3-K, Akt, and mTOR. *Future Neurol.* 7:733-748

Chong, Z. Z., Shang, Y. C., Wang, S., Maiese, K. (2012b) PRAS40 is an integral regulatory component of erythropoietin mTOR signaling and cytoprotection. *PLoS One* 7:e45456

Chong, Z. Z., Shang, Y. C., Wang, S., Maiese, K. (2012c) Shedding new light on neurodegenerative diseases through the mammalian target of rapamycin. *Prog. Neurobiol.* 99:128-148

Chong, Z. Z., Shang, Y. C., Zhang, L., Wang, S., Maiese, K. (2010b) Mammalian target of rapamycin: hitting the bull's-eye for neurological disorders. *Oxid. Med. Cell Longev.* 3:374-391

Chong, Z. Z., Yao, Q., Li, H. H. (2013) The rationale of targeting mammalian target of rapamycin for ischemic stroke. *Cell Signal*

Coladonato, J. A., Frankenfield, D. L., Reddan, D. N., Klassen, P. S., Szczech, L. A., Johnson, C. A., Owen, W. F., Jr. (2002) Trends in anemia management among US hemodialysis patients. *J. Am. Soc. Nephrol.* 13: 1288-1295

Crivellato, E., Nico, B., Vacca, A., Djonov, V., Presta, M., Ribatti, D. (2004) Recombinant human erythropoietin induces intussusceptive microvascular growth in vivo. *Leukemia* 18:331-336

Dame, C., Fahnenstich, H., Freitag, P., Hofmann, D., Abdul-Nour, T., Bartmann, P., Fandrey, J. (1998) Erythropoietin mRNA expression in human fetal and neonatal tissue. *Blood* 92:3218-3225

Danielyan, L., Schafer, R., Schulz, A., Ladewig, T., Lourhmati, A., Buadze, M., Schmitt, A. L., Verleysdonk, S., Kabisch, D., Koeppen, K., Siegel, G., Proksch, B., Kluba, T., Eckert, A., Kohle, C., Schoneberg, T., Northoff, H., Schwab, M., Gleiter, C. H. (2009) Survival, neuron-like differentiation and functionality of mesenchymal stem cells in neurotoxic environment: the critical role of erythropoietin. *Cell Death Differ.* 16:1599-1614

Das, M., Scappini, E., Martin, N. P., Wong, K. A., Dunn, S., Chen, Y. J., Miller, S. L., Domin, J., O'Bryan, J. P. (2007) Regulation of neuron survival through an intersectin-phosphoinositide 3'-kinase C2beta-AKT pathway. *Mol. Cell Biol.* 27:7906-7917

De Smaele, E., Zazzeroni, F., Papa, S., Nguyen, D. U., Jin, R., Jones, J., Cong, R., Franzoso, G. (2001) Induction of gadd45beta by NF-kappaB downregulates pro-apoptotic JNK signalling. *Nature* 414:308-313

Digicaylioglu, M., Bichet, S., Marti, H. H., Wenger, R. H., Rivas, L. A., Bauer, C., Gassmann, M. (1995) Localization of specific erythropoietin binding sites in defined areas of the mouse brain. *Proc. Natl. Acad. Sci. US* 92:3717-3720.

Digicaylioglu, M., Lipton, S. A. (2001) Erythropoietin-mediated neuroprotection involves cross-talk between Jak2 and NF-kappaB signalling cascades. *Nature* 412:641-647.

Drueke, T. B., Locatelli, F., Clyne, N., Eckardt, K. U., Macdougall, I. C., Tsakiris, D., Burger, H. U., Scherhag, A. (2006) Normalization of hemoglobin level in patients with chronic kidney disease and anemia. *N Engl. J. Med.* 355:2071-2084

Dube, S., Fisher, J. W., Powell, J. S. (1988) Glycosylation at specific sites of erythropoietin is essential for biosynthesis, secretion, and biological function. *J. Biol. Chem.* 263:17516-17521.

Dzietko, M., Felderhoff-Mueser, U., Sifringer, M., Krutz, B., Bittigau, P., Thor, F., Heumann, R., Buhrer, C., Ikonomidou, C., Hansen, H. H. (2004) Erythropoietin protects the developing brain against N-methyl-D-aspartate receptor antagonist neurotoxicity. *Neurobiol. Dis.* 15:177-187

Erbayraktar, S., Grasso, G., Sfacteria, A., Xie, Q. W., Coleman, T., Kreilgaard, M., Torup, L., Sager, T., Erbayraktar, Z., Gokmen, N., Yilmaz, O., Ghezzi, P., Villa, P., Fratelli, M., Casagrande, S., Leist, M., Helboe, L., Gerwein, J., Christensen, S., Geist, M. A., Pedersen, L. O., Cerami-Hand, C., Wuerth, J. P., Cerami, A., Brines, M. (2003) Asialoerythropoietin is a nonerythropoietic cytokine with broad neuroprotective activity in vivo. *Proc. Natl. Acad. Sci. US* 100:6741-6746

Eschbach, J. W., Egrie, J. C., Downing, M. R., Browne, J. K., Adamson, J. W. (1987) Correction of the anemia of end-stage renal disease with recombinant human erythropoietin. Results of a combined phase I and II clinical trial. *N Engl. J. Med.* 316:73-78

Eschbach, J. W., Haley, N. R., Adamson, J. W. (1989) The use of recombinant erythropoietin in the treatment of the anemia of chronic renal failure. *Ann. N Y Acad. Sci.* 554:225-230

Fan, X., Heijnen, C. J., van der, K. M., Groenendaal, F., van Bel, F. (2011) Beneficial effect of erythropoietin on sensorimotor function and white matter after hypoxia-ischemia in neonatal mice. *Pediatr. Res.* 69:56-61

Feng, G. S., Shen, R., Heng, H. H., Tsui, L. C., Kazlauskas, A., Pawson, T. (1994) Receptor-binding, tyrosine phosphorylation and chromosome localization of the mouse SH2-containing phosphotyrosine phosphatase Syp. *Oncogene* 9:1545-1550

Ferrario, M., Arbustini, E., Massa, M., Rosti, V., Marziliano, N., Raineri, C., Campanelli, R., Bertoletti, A., De Ferrari, G. M., Klersy, C., Angoli, L., Bramucci, E., Marinoni, B., Ferlini, M., Moretti, E., Raisaro, A., Repetto, A., Schwartz, P. J., Tavazzi, L. (2011) High-dose erythropoietin in patients with acute myocardial infarction: a pilot, randomised, placebo-controlled study. *Int. J. Cardiol.* 147:124-131

Fisher, J. W. (2003) Erythropoietin: physiology and pharmacology update. *Exp. Biol. Med. (Maywood)* 228:1-14

Fisher, J. W., Birdwell, B. J. (1961) The production of an erythropoietic factor by the in situ perfused kidney. *Acta Haematol.* 26:224-232

Gabel, R., Klopsch, C., Furlani, D., Yerebakan, C., Li, W., Ugurlucan, M., Ma, N., Steinhoff, G. (2009) Single high-dose intramyocardial administration of erythropoietin promotes early intracardiac proliferation, proves safety and restores cardiac performance after myocardial infarction in rats. *Interact. Cardiovasc. Thorac. Surg.* 9:20-25; discussion 25

Galson, D. L., Tsuchiya, T., Tendler, D. S., Huang, L. E., Ren, Y., Ogura, T., Bunn, H. F. (1995) The orphan receptor hepatic nuclear factor 4 functions as a transcriptional activator for tissue-specific and hypoxia-specific erythropoietin gene expression and is antagonized by EAR3/COUP-TF1. *Mol. Cell. Biol.* 15:2135-2144

Gao, D., Ning, N., Niu, X., Dang, Y., Dong, X., Wei, J., Zhu, C. (2012) Erythropoietin treatment in patients with acute myocardial infarction: a meta-analysis of randomized controlled trials. *Am. Heart J.* 164:715-727 e711

Genc, S., Koroglu, T. F., Genc, K. (2004) Erythropoietin and the nervous system. *Brain Res.* 1000:19-31

Gobert, S., Chretien, S., Gouilleux, F., Muller, O., Pallard, C., Dusanter-Fourt, I., Groner, B., Lacombe, C., Gisselbrecht, S., Mayeux, P. (1996) Identification of tyrosine residues within the intracellular domain of the erythropoietin receptor crucial for STAT5 activation. *Embo J.* 15:2434-2441.

Goldberg, N., Lundin, A. P., Delano, B., Friedman, E. A., Stein, R. A. (1992) Changes in left ventricular size, wall thickness, and function in anemic patients treated with recombinant human erythropoietin. *Am. Heart J.* 124: 424-427

Gonzalez, F. F., McQuillen, P., Mu, D., Chang, Y., Wendland, M., Vexler, Z., Ferriero, D. M. (2007) Erythropoietin enhances long-term neuroprotection and neurogenesis in neonatal stroke. *Dev. Neurosci.* 29:321-330

Grunfeld, J. F., Barhum, Y., Blondheim, N., Rabey, J. M., Melamed, E., Offen, D. (2007) Erythropoietin delays disease onset in an amyotrophic lateral sclerosis model. *Exp. Neurol.* 204:260-263

Hagemeyer, N., Boretius, S., Ott, C., Von Streitberg, A., Welpinghus, H., Sperling, S., Frahm, J., Simons, M., Ghezzi, P., Ehrenreich, H. (2012) Erythropoietin attenuates neurological and histological consequences of toxic demyelination in mice. *Mol. Med.* 18:628-635

Hale, S. L., Sesti, C., Kloner, R. A. (2005) Administration of erythropoietin fails to improve long-term healing or cardiac function after myocardial infarction in the rat. *J. Cardiovasc. Pharmacol.* 46:211-215

Hanahan, D., Folkman, J. (1996) Patterns and emerging mechanisms of the angiogenic switch during tumorigenesis. *Cell* 86:353-364.

Hand, M. F., Haynes, W. G., Johnstone, H. A., Anderton, J. L., Webb, D. J. (1995) Erythropoietin enhances vascular responsiveness to norepinephrine in renal failure. *Kidney Int.* 48:806-813.

Hiort, E. (1936) Reticulocyte increase after injection of anemic serum. *Mag. F Laegividensk* 97:270-277

Hirata, A., Minamino, T., Asanuma, H., Fujita, M., Wakeno, M., Myoishi, M., Tsukamoto, O., Okada, K., Koyama, H., Komamura, K., Takashima, S., Shinozaki, Y., Mori, H., Shiraga, M., Kitakaze, M., Hori, M. (2006) Erythropoietin enhances neovascularization of ischemic myocardium and improves left ventricular dysfunction after myocardial infarction in dogs. *J. Am. Coll Cardiol.* 48:176-184

Hoffman, E. C., Reyes, H., Chu, F. F., Sander, F., Conley, L. H., Brooks, B. A., Hankinson, O. (1991) Cloning of a factor required for activity of the Ah (dioxin) receptor. *Science* 252:954-958.

Hou, J., Chong, Z. Z., Shang, Y. C., Maiese, K. (2010) FOXO3a governs early and late apoptotic endothelial programs during elevated glucose through mitochondrial and caspase signaling. *Mol. Cell Endocrinol.* 321:194-206

Hou, J., Wang, S., Shang, Y. C., Chong, Z. Z., Maiese, K. (2011) Erythropoietin Employs Cell Longevity Pathways of SIRT1 to Foster Endothelial Vascular Integrity During Oxidant Stress. *Curr. Neurovasc. Res.*

Huang, L. E., Gu, J., Schau, M., Bunn, H. F. (1998) Regulation of hypoxia-inducible factor 1alpha is mediated by an O2- dependent degradation domain via the ubiquitin-proteasome pathway. *Proc. Natl. Acad. Sci. US* 95:7987-7992.

Imai, N., Kawamura, A., Higuchi, M., Oh-eda, M., Orita, T., Kawaguchi, T., Ochi, N. (1990) Physicochemical and biological comparison of recombinant human erythropoietin with human urinary erythropoietin. *J. Biochem. (Tokyo)* 107:352-359.

Ivan, M., Kondo, K., Yang, H., Kim, W., Valiando, J., Ohh, M., Salic, A., Asara, J. M., Lane, W. S., Kaelin, W. G., Jr. (2001) HIFalpha targeted for VHL-mediated destruction by proline hydroxylation: implications for O2 sensing. *Science* 292:464-468

Jaakkola, P., Mole, D. R., Tian, Y. M., Wilson, M. I., Gielbert, J., Gaskell, S. J., von Kriegsheim, A., Hebestreit, H. F., Mukherji, M., Schofield, C. J., Maxwell, P. H., Pugh, C. W., Ratcliffe, P. J. (2001) Targeting of HIF-alpha to the von Hippel-Lindau ubiquitylation complex by O2-regulated prolyl hydroxylation. *Science* 292:468-472

Jacobs, K., Shoemaker, C., Rudersdorf, R., Neill, S. D., Kaufman, R. J., Mufson, A., Seehra, J., Jones, S. S., Hewick, R., Fritsch, E. F., et al. (1985) Isolation and characterization of genomic and cDNA clones of human erythropoietin. *Nature* 313:806-810.

Jacobs-Helber, S. M., Ryan, J. J., Sawyer, S. T. (2000) JNK and p38 are activated by erythropoietin (EPO) but are not induced in apoptosis following EPO withdrawal in EPO-dependent HCD57 cells. *Blood* 96: 933-940.

Jacobson, L. O., Goldwasser, E., Fried, W., Plzak, L. (1957) Role of the kidney in erythropoiesis. *Nature* 179:633-634

Janik, P., Kwiecinski, H., Sokolowska, B., Niebroj-Dobosz, I. (2010) Erythropoietin concentration in serum and cerebrospinal fluid of patients with amyotrophic lateral sclerosis. *J. Neural Transm.* 117:343-347

Jelkmann, W., Bauer, C. (1981) Demonstration of high levels of erythropoietin in rat kidneys following hypoxic hypoxia. *Pflugers Arch.* 392:34-39

Jung, K. H., Chu, K., Lee, S. T., Park, K. I., Kim, J. H., Kang, K. M., Kim, S., Jeon, D., Kim, M., Lee, S. K., Roh, J. K. (2011) Molecular alterations underlying epileptogenesis after prolonged febrile seizure and modulation by erythropoietin. *Epilepsia* 52:541-550

Juul, S. E., Yachnis, A. T., Rojiani, A. M., Christensen, R. D. (1999) Immunohistochemical localization of erythropoietin and its receptor in the developing human brain. *Pediatr. Dev. Pathol.* 2:148-158.

Kadota, T., Shingo, T., Yasuhara, T., Tajiri, N., Kondo, A., Morimoto, T., Yuan, W. J., Wang, F., Baba, T., Tokunaga, K., Miyoshi, Y., Date, I. (2009) Continuous intraventricular infusion of erythropoietin exerts neuroprotective/rescue effects upon Parkinson's disease model of rats with enhanced neurogenesis. *Brain Res.* 1254:120-127

Kanaan, N. M., Collier, T. J., Marchionini, D. M., McGuire, S. O., Fleming, M. F., Sortwell, C. E. (2006) Exogenous erythropoietin provides neuroprotection of grafted dopamine neurons in a rodent model of Parkinson's disease. *Brain Res.* 1068:221-229

Kato, S., Aoyama, M., Kakita, H., Hida, H., Kato, I., Ito, T., Goto, T., Hussein, M. H., Sawamoto, K., Togari, H., Asai, K. (2011) Endogenous erythropoietin from astrocyte protects the oligodendrocyte precursor cell against hypoxic and reoxygenation injury. *J. Neurosci. Res.* 89:1566-1574

Kaupke, C. J., Kim, S., Vaziri, N. D. (1994) Effect of erythrocyte mass on arterial blood pressure in dialysis patients receiving maintenance erythropoietin therapy. *J. Am. Soc. Nephrol.* 4:1874-1878.

Kim, J. E., Chen, J., Lou, Z. (2008) DBC1 is a negative regulator of SIRT1. *Nature* 451:583-586

Klingmuller, U., Lorenz, U., Cantley, L. C., Neel, B. G., Lodish, H. F. (1995) Specific recruitment of SH-PTP1 to the erythropoietin receptor causes inactivation of JAK2 and termination of proliferative signals. *Cell* 80:729-738

Koh, S. H., Kim, Y., Kim, H. Y., Cho, G. W., Kim, K. S., Kim, S. H. (2007) Recombinant human erythropoietin suppresses symptom onset and progression of G93A-SOD1 mouse model of ALS by preventing motor neuron death and inflammation. *Eur. J. Neurosci.* 25:1923-1930

Kondo, A., Shingo, T., Yasuhara, T., Kuramoto, S., Kameda, M., Kikuchi, Y., Matsui, T., Miyoshi, Y., Agari, T., Borlongan, C. V., Date, I. (2009) Erythropoietin exerts anti-epileptic effects with the suppression of aberrant new cell formation in the dentate gyrus and upregulation of neuropeptide Y in seizure model of rats. *Brain Res.* 1296:127-136

Kook, Y. H., Ka, M., Um, M. (2011) Neuroprotective cytokines repress PUMA induction in the 1-methyl-4-phenylpyridinium (MPP(+)) model of Parkinson's disease. *Biochem. Biophys. Res. Commun.* 411:370-374

Krantz, S. B. (1990) Review of patients' responses to epoetin alfa therapy. *Pharmacotherapy* 10:15S-21S

Krantz, S. B. (1991) Erythropoietin. *Blood* 77:419-434.

Krumdieck, N. (1943) Erythropoietic substance in the serum of anemic animals. *Proc. Exp. Biol. Med.* 54:15-17

Kuratowska, Z., Lewartowski, B., Michalak, E. (1961) Studies on the production of erythropoietin by isolated perfused organs. *Blood* 18:527-534

Kyriakis, J. M. (2001) Life-or-death decisions. *Nature* 414:265-266.

Lando, D., Peet, D. J., Gorman, J. J., Whelan, D. A., Whitelaw, M. L., Bruick, R. K. (2002) FIH-1 is an asparaginyl hydroxylase enzyme that regulates the transcriptional activity of hypoxia-inducible factor. *Genes Dev.* 16:1466-1471

Lebel, M., Kingma, I., Grose, J. H., Langlois, S. (1998) Hemodynamic and hormonal changes during erythropoietin therapy in hemodialysis patients. *J. Am. Soc. Nephrol.* 9:97-104.

Leconte, C., Bihel, E., Lepelletier, F. X., Bouet, V., Saulnier, R., Petit, E., Boulouard, M., Bernaudin, M., Schumann-Bard, P. (2011) Comparison of the effects of erythropoietin and its carbamylated derivative on behaviour and hippocampal neurogenesis in mice. *Neuropharmacology* 60:354-364

Lee, C. W., Wong, L. L., Tse, E. Y., Liu, H. F., Leong, V. Y., Lee, J. M., Hardie, D. G., Ng, I. O., Ching, Y. P. (2012) AMPK promotes p53 acetylation via phosphorylation and inactivation of SIRT1 in liver cancer cells. *Cancer Res.* 72:4394-4404

Leist, M., Ghezzi, P., Grasso, G., Bianchi, R., Villa, P., Fratelli, M., Savino, C., Bianchi, M., Nielsen, J., Gerwien, J., Kallunki, P., Larsen, A. K., Helboe, L., Christensen, S., Pedersen, L. O., Nielsen, M., Torup, L., Sager, T., Sfacteria, A., Erbayraktar, S., Erbayraktar, Z., Gokmen, N., Yilmaz, O., Cerami-Hand, C., Xie, Q. W., Coleman, T., Cerami, A., Brines, M. (2004) Derivatives of erythropoietin that are tissue protective but not erythropoietic. *Science* 305:239-242

Li, F., Chong, Z. Z., Maiese, K. (2006) Microglial integrity is maintained by erythropoietin through integration of Akt and its substrates of glycogen synthase kinase-3beta, beta-catenin, and nuclear factor-kappaB. *Curr. Neurovasc. Res.* 3:187-201

Li, Y., Lu, Z., Keogh, C. L., Yu, S. P., Wei, L. (2007) Erythropoietin-induced neurovascular protection, angiogenesis, and cerebral blood flow restoration after focal ischemia in mice. *J. Cereb. Blood Flow Metab.* 27: 1043-1054

Lin, F. K., Suggs, S., Lin, C. H., Browne, J. K., Smalling, R., Egrie, J. C., Chen, K. K., Fox, G. M., Martin, F., Stabinsky, Z., et al. (1985) Cloning and expression of the human erythropoietin gene. *Proc. Natl. Acad. Sci. US* 82:7580-7584

Littlewood, T. J. (2001) Erythropoietin for the treatment of anemia associated with hematological malignancy. *Hematol. Oncol.* 19:19-30.

Liu, D., Wen, J., Liu, J., Li, L. (1999) The roles of free radicals in amyotrophic lateral sclerosis: reactive oxygen species and elevated oxidation of protein, DNA, and membrane phospholipids. *Faseb J.* 13:2318-2328.

Liu, R., Suzuki, A., Guo, Z., Mizuno, Y., Urabe, T. (2006) Intrinsic and extrinsic erythropoietin enhances neuroprotection against ischemia and reperfusion injury in vitro. *J. Neurochem.* 96:1101-1110

Low-Friedrich, I., Grutzmacher, P., Marz, W., Bergmann, M., Schoeppe, W. (1991) Therapy with recombinant human erythropoietin reduces cardiac size and improves heart function in chronic hemodialysis patients. *Am. J. Nephrol.* 11:54-60

Lui, S. F., Chung, W. W., Leung, C. B., Chan, K., Lai, K. N. (1990) Pharmacokinetics and pharmacodynamics of subcutaneous and intraperitoneal administration of recombinant human erythropoietin in patients on continuous ambulatory peritoneal dialysis. *Clin. Nephrol.* 33: 47-51

Ma, R., Xiong, N., Huang, C., Tang, Q., Hu, B., Xiang, J., Li, G. (2009) Erythropoietin protects PC12 cells from beta-amyloid(25-35)-induced apoptosis via PI3K/Akt signaling pathway. *Neuropharmacology* 56:1027-1034

Mahmud, D. L., M. G. A., Deb, D. K., Platanias, L. C., Uddin, S., Wickrema, A. (2002) Phosphorylation of forkhead transcription factors by erythropoietin and stem cell factor prevents acetylation and their interaction with coactivator p300 in erythroid progenitor cells. *Oncogene* 21:1556-1562

Maiese, K. (2008) Triple play: promoting neurovascular longevity with nicotinamide, WNT, and erythropoietin in diabetes mellitus. *Biomed. Pharmacother.* 62:218-232

Maiese, K., Li, F., Chong, Z. Z. (2004) Erythropoietin in the brain: can the promise to protect be fulfilled? *Trends Pharmacol. Sci.* 25:577-583

Marti, H. H. (2004) Erythropoietin and the hypoxic brain. *J. Exp. Biol.* 207: 3233-3242

Marti, H. H., Gassmann, M., Wenger, R. H., Kvietikova, I., Morganti-Kossmann, M. C., Kossmann, T., Trentz, O., Bauer, C. (1997) Detection of erythropoietin in human liquor: intrinsic erythropoietin production in the brain. *Kidney Int.* 51:416-418.

Marti, H. H., Wenger, R. H., Rivas, L. A., Straumann, U., Digicaylioglu, M., Henn, V., Yonekawa, Y., Bauer, C., Gassmann, M. (1996) Erythropoietin gene expression in human, monkey and murine brain. *Eur. J. Neurosci.* 8: 666-676.

Masuda, S., Kobayashi, T., Chikuma, M., Nagao, M., Sasaki, R. (2000) The oviduct produces erythropoietin in an estrogen- and oxygen- dependent manner. *Am. J. Physiol. Endocrinol. Metab.* 278:E1038-1044.

Masuda, S., Nagao, M., Takahata, K., Konishi, Y., Gallyas, F., Jr., Tabira, T., Sasaki, R. (1993) Functional erythropoietin receptor of the cells with neural characteristics. Comparison with receptor properties of erythroid cells. *J. Biol. Chem.* 268:11208-11216.

Masuda, S., Okano, M., Yamagishi, K., Nagao, M., Ueda, M., Sasaki, R. (1994) A novel site of erythropoietin production. Oxygen-dependent production in cultured rat astrocytes. *J. Biol. Chem.* 269:19488-19493.

Matsuzaki, H., Tamatani, M., Mitsuda, N., Namikawa, K., Kiyama, H., Miyake, S., Tohyama, M. (1999) Activation of Akt kinase inhibits apoptosis and changes in Bcl-2 and Bax expression induced by nitric oxide in primary hippocampal neurons. *J. Neurochem.* 73:2037-2046.

Mikati, M. A., El Hokayem, J. A., El Sabban, M. E. (2007) Effects of a single dose of erythropoietin on subsequent seizure susceptibility in rats exposed to acute hypoxia at P10. *Epilepsia* 48:175-181

Milarski, K. L., Saltiel, A. R. (1994) Expression of catalytically inactive Syp phosphatase in 3T3 cells blocks stimulation of mitogen-activated protein kinase by insulin. *J. Biol. Chem.* 269:21239-21243

Miyake, T., Kung, C. K., Goldwasser, E. (1977) Purification of human erythropoietin. *J. Biol. Chem.* 252:5558-5564

Moon, C., Krawczyk, M., Ahn, D., Ahmet, I., Paik, D., Lakatta, E. G., Talan, M. I. (2003) Erythropoietin reduces myocardial infarction and left ventricular functional decline after coronary artery ligation in rats. *Proc. Natl. Acad. Sci. US* 100:11612-11617

Moon, C., Krawczyk, M., Paik, D., Coleman, T., Brines, M., Juhaszova, M., Sollott, S. J., Lakatta, E. G., Talan, M. I. (2006) Erythropoietin, modified to not stimulate red blood cell production, retains its cardioprotective properties. *J. Pharmacol. Exp. Ther.* 316:999-1005

Moon, C., Krawczyk, M., Paik, D., Lakatta, E. G., Talan, M. I. (2005) Cardioprotection by recombinant human erythropoietin following acute experimental myocardial infarction: dose response and therapeutic window. *Cardiovasc. Drugs Ther.* 19:243-250

Moran, L. J., Carey, P., Johnson, C. A. (1992) Cost-effectiveness of epoetin alfa therapy for anemia of end-stage renal disease. *Am. J. Hosp. Pharm.* 49:1451-1454

Morishita, E., Masuda, S., Nagao, M., Yasuda, Y., Sasaki, R. (1997) Erythropoietin receptor is expressed in rat hippocampal and cerebral cortical neurons, and erythropoietin prevents in vitro glutamate- induced neuronal death. *Neuroscience* 76:105-116.

Mukundan, H., Resta, T. C., Kanagy, N. L. (2002) 17Beta-estradiol decreases hypoxic induction of erythropoietin gene expression. *Am. J. Physiol. Regul. Integr. Comp. Physiol.* 283:R496-504

Mulcahy, L. (2001) The erythropoietin receptor. *Semin. Oncol.* 28:19-23.

Naganska, E., Taraszewska, A., Matyja, E., Grieb, P., Rafalowska, J. (2010) Neuroprotective effect of erythropoietin in amyotrophic lateral sclerosis (ALS) model in vitro. Ultrastructural study. *Folia Neuropathol.* 48:35-44

Najjar, S. S., Rao, S. V., Melloni, C., Raman, S. V., Povsic, T. J., Melton, L., Barsness, G. W., Prather, K., Heitner, J. F., Kilaru, R., Gruberg, L., Hasselblad, V., Greenbaum, A. B., Patel, M., Kim, R. J., Talan, M., Ferrucci, .L, Longo, D. L., Lakatta, E. G., Harrington, R. A. (2011) Intravenous erythropoietin in patients with ST-segment elevation myocardial infarction: REVEAL: a randomized controlled trial. *Jama* 305: 1863-1872

Namiuchi, S., Kagaya, Y., Ohta, J., Shiba, N., Sugi, M., Oikawa, M., Kunii, H., Yamao, H., Komatsu, N., Yui, M., Tada, H., Sakuma, M., Watanabe, J., Ichihara, T., Shirato, K. (2005) High serum erythropoietin level is associated with smaller infarct size in patients with acute myocardial infarction who undergo successful primary percutaneous coronary intervention. *J. Am. Coll Cardiol.* 45:1406-1412

Nascimento, E. B., Snel, M., Guigas, B., van der Zon, G. C., Kriek, J., Maassen, J. A., Jazet, I. M., Diamant, M., Ouwens, D. M. (2010)

Phosphorylation of PRAS40 on Thr246 by PKB/AKT facilitates efficient phosphorylation of Ser183 by mTORC1. *Cell Signal.* 22:961-967

Nguyen, M. H., Ho, J. M., Beattie, B. K., Barber, D. L. (2001) TEL-JAK2 mediates constitutive activation of the phosphatidylinositol 3'-kinase/protein kinase B signaling pathway. *J. Biol. Chem.* 276:32704-32713.

Ogawa, A., Terada, S., Sakuragawa, N., Masuda, S., Nagao, M., Miki, M. (2003) Progesterone, but not 17beta-estradiol, up-regulates erythropoietin (EPO) production in human amniotic epithelial cells. *J. Biosci. Bioeng.* 96:448-453

Pandey, M. K., Sung, B., Ahn, K. S., Aggarwal, B. B. (2009) Butein suppresses constitutive and inducible signal transducer and activator of transcription (STAT) 3 activation and STAT3-regulated gene products through the induction of a protein tyrosine phosphatase SHP-1. *Mol. Pharmacol.* 75:525-533

Park, K. H., Choi, N. Y., Koh, S. H., Park, H. H., Kim, Y. S., Kim, M. J., Lee, S. J., Yu, H. J., Lee, K. Y., Lee, Y. J., Kim, H. T. (2011) L-DOPA neurotoxicity is prevented by neuroprotective effects of erythropoietin. *Neurotoxicology* 32:879-887

Parsa, C. J., Kim, J., Riel, R. U., Pascal, L. S., Thompson, R. B., Petrofski, J. A., Matsumoto, A., Stamler, J. S., Koch, W. J. (2004) Cardioprotective effects of erythropoietin in the reperfused ischemic heart: a potential role for cardiac fibroblasts. *J. Biol. Chem.*

Parsa, C. J., Matsumoto, A., Kim, J., Riel, R. U., Pascal, L. S., Walton, G. B., Thompson, R. B., Petrofski, J. A., Annex, B. H., Stamler, J. S., Koch, W. J. (2003) A novel protective effect of erythropoietin in the infarcted heart. *J. Clin. Invest.* 112:999-1007

Reed, J. C. (2001) Apoptosis-regulating proteins as targets for drug discovery. *Trends Mol. Med.* 7:314-319.

Ribatti, D., Presta, M., Vacca, A., Ria, R., Giuliani, R., Dell'Era, P., Nico, B., Roncali, L., Dammacco, F. (1999) Human erythropoietin induces a pro-angiogenic phenotype in cultured endothelial cells and stimulates neovascularization in vivo. *Blood* 93:2627-2636.

Risau, W. (1997) Mechanisms of angiogenesis. *Nature* 386:671-674.

Roger, S. D., Grasty, M. S., Baker, L. R., Raine, A. E. (1992) Effects of oxygen breathing and erythropoietin on hypoxic vasodilation in uremic anemia. *Kidney Int.* 42:975-980.

Sandor, G. (1932) Uber die blutbildende Wirkung des Serums von Tieren, die in verdunnter Luft gehalten wurden. *Z Ges. Exp. Med.* 82:636-646

Sasaki, H., Bothner, B., Dell, A., Fukuda, M. (1987) Carbohydrate structure of erythropoietin expressed in Chinese hamster ovary cells by a human erythropoietin cDNA. *J. Biol. Chem.* 262:12059-12076.

Savino, C., Pedotti, R., Baggi, F., Ubiali, F., Gallo, B., Nava, S., Bigini, P., Barbera, S., Fumagalli, E., Mennini, T., Vezzani, A., Rizzi, M., Coleman, T., Cerami, A., Brines, M., Ghezzi, P., Bianchi, R. (2006) Delayed administration of erythropoietin and its non-erythropoietic derivatives ameliorates chronic murine autoimmune encephalomyelitis. *J. Neuroimmunol.* 172:27-37

Schaefer, R. M., Leschke, M., Strauer, B. E., Heidland, A. (1988) Blood rheology and hypertension in hemodialysis patients treated with erythropoietin. *Am. J. Nephrol.* 8:449-453

Semenza, G. L. (2004) O2-regulated gene expression: transcriptional control of cardiorespiratory physiology by HIF-1. *J. Appl. Physiol.* 96:1173-1177; discussion 1170-1172

Shang, Y., Wu, Y., Yao, S., Wang, X., Feng, D., Yang, W. (2007) Protective effect of erythropoietin against ketamine-induced apoptosis in cultured rat cortical neurons: involvement of PI3K/Akt and GSK-3 beta pathway. *Apoptosis* 12:2187-2195

Shang, Y. C., Chong, Z. Z., Hou, J., Maiese, K. (2009a) FoxO3a governs early microglial proliferation and employs mitochondrial depolarization with caspase 3, 8, and 9 cleavage during oxidant induced apoptosis. *Curr. Neurovasc. Res.* 6:223-238

Shang, Y. C., Chong, Z. Z., Hou, J., Maiese, K. (2009b) The forkhead transcription factor FOXO3a controls microglial inflammatory activation and eventual apoptotic injury through caspase 3. *Curr. Neurovasc. Res.* 6: 20-31

Shang, Y. C., Chong, Z. Z., Hou, J., Maiese, K. (2010) Wnt1, FoxO3a, and NF-kappaB oversee microglial integrity and activation during oxidant stress. *Cell Signal* 22:1317-1329

Shang, Y. C., Chong, Z. Z., Wang, S., Maiese, K. (2011) Erythropoietin and Wnt1 Govern Pathways of mTOR, Apaf-1, and XIAP in Inflammatory Microglia. *Curr. Neurovasc. Res.*

Shang, Y. C., Chong, Z. Z., Wang, S., Maiese, K. (2012) Prevention of beta-amyloid degeneration of microglia by erythropoietin depends on Wnt1, the PI 3-K/mTOR pathway, Bad, and Bcl-xL. *Aging (Albany NY)* 4:187-201

Shen, J., Wu, Y., Xu, J. Y., Zhang, J., Sinclair, S. H., Yanoff, M., Xu, G., Li, W., Xu, G. T. (2010) ERK- and Akt-dependent neuroprotection by erythropoietin (EPO) against glyoxal-AGEs via modulation of Bcl-xL, Bax, and BAD. *Invest. Ophthalmol. Vis. Sci.* 51:35-46

Shingo, T., Sorokan, S. T., Shimazaki, T., Weiss, S. (2001) Erythropoietin regulates the in vitro and in vivo production of neuronal progenitors by mammalian forebrain neural stem cells. *J. Neurosci.* 21:9733-9743.

Signore, A. P., Weng, Z., Hastings, T., Van Laar, A. D., Liang, Q., Lee, Y. J., Chen, J. (2006) Erythropoietin protects against 6-hydroxydopamine-induced dopaminergic cell death. *J. Neurochem.* 96:428-443

Silverberg, D. S., Wexler, D., Blum, M., Tchebiner, J. Z., Sheps, D., Keren, G., Schwartz, D., Baruch, R., Yachnin, T., Shaked, M., Schwartz, I., Steinbruch, S., Iaina, A. (2003) The effect of correction of anaemia in diabetics and non-diabetics with severe resistant congestive heart failure and chronic renal failure by subcutaneous erythropoietin and intravenous iron. *Nephrol. Dial. Transplant.* 18:141-146

Silverberg, D. S., Wexler, D., Sheps, D., Blum, M., Keren, G., Baruch, R., Schwartz, D., Yachnin, T., Steinbruch, S., Shapira, I., Laniado, S., Iaina, A. (2001) The effect of correction of mild anemia in severe, resistant congestive heart failure using subcutaneous erythropoietin and intravenous iron: a randomized controlled study. *J. Am. Coll Cardiol.* 37: 1775-1780

Singh, N. P., Sahni, V., Wadhwa, A., Garg, S., Bajaj, S. K., Kohli, R., Agarwal, S. K. (2006) Effect of improvement in anemia on electroneurophysiological markers (P300) of cognitive dysfunction in chronic kidney disease. *Hemodial. Int.* 10:267-273

Socolovsky, M., Fallon, A. E., Wang, S., Brugnara, C., Lodish, H. F. (1999) Fetal anemia and apoptosis of red cell progenitors in Stat5a-/-5b-/- mice: a direct role for Stat5 in Bcl-X(L) induction. *Cell* 98:181-191.

Sozmen, S. C., Kurul, S. H., Yis, U., Tugyan, K., Baykara, B., Yilmaz, O. (2012) Neuroprotective effects of recombinant human erythropoietin in the developing brain of rat after lithium-pilocarpine induced status epilepticus. *Brain Dev.* 34:189-195

Steffen, H. M., Brunner, R., Muller, R., Degenhardt, S., Pollok, M., Lang, R., Baldamus, C. A. (1989) Peripheral hemodynamics, blood viscosity, and the renin-angiotensin system in hemodialysis patients under therapy with recombinant human erythropoietin. *Contrib. Nephrol.* 76:292-298

Stephens, L., Anderson, K., Stokoe, D., Erdjument-Bromage, H., Painter, G. F., Holmes, A. B., Gaffney, P. R., Reese, C. B., McCormick, F., Tempst, P., Coadwell, J., Hawkins, P. T. (1998) Protein kinase B kinases that mediate phosphatidylinositol 3,4,5-trisphosphate-dependent activation of protein kinase B. *Science* 279:710-714

Sun, Z. K., Yang, H. Q., Pan, J., Zhen, H., Wang, Z. Q., Chen, S. D., Ding, J. Q. (2008) Protective effects of erythropoietin on tau phosphorylation induced by beta-amyloid. *J. Neurosci. Res.* 86:3018-3027

Suzuki, T., Sasaki, R. (1990) Immunocytochemical demonstration of erythropoietin immunoreactivity in peritubular endothelial cells of the anemic mouse kidney. *Arch. Histol. Cytol.* 53:121-124

Tang, H., Chen, S., Wang, H., Wu, H., Lu, Q., Han, D. (2009) TAM receptors and the regulation of erythropoiesis in mice. *Haematologica* 94:326-334

Tang, K., Yang, J., Gao, X., Wang, C., Liu, L., Kitani, H., Atsumi, T., Jing, N. (2002) Wnt-1 promotes neuronal differentiation and inhibits gliogenesis in P19 cells. *Biochem. Biophys. Res. Commun.* 293:167-173.

Toyoda, T., Itai, T., Arakawa, T., Aoki, K. H., Yamaguchi, H. (2000) Stabilization of human recombinant erythropoietin through interactions with the highly branched N-glycans. *J. Biochem. (Tokyo)* 128:731-737.

Tramontano, A. F., Muniyappa, R., Black, A. D., Blendea, M. C., Cohen, I., Deng, L., Sowers, J. R., Cutaia, M. V., El-Sherif, N. (2003) Erythropoietin protects cardiac myocytes from hypoxia-induced apoptosis through an Akt-dependent pathway. *Biochem. Biophys. Res. Commun.* 308:990-994

Tsuda, E., Goto, M., Murakami, A., Akai, K., Ueda, M., Kawanishi, G., Takahashi, N., Sasaki, R., Chiba, H., Ishihara, H., et al. (1988) Comparative structural study of N-linked oligosaccharides of urinary and recombinant erythropoietins. *Biochemistry* 27:5646-5654.

Uchida, E., Morimoto, K., Kawasaki, N., Izaki, Y., Abdu Said, A., Hayakawa, T. (1997) Effect of active oxygen radicals on protein and carbohydrate moieties of recombinant human erythropoietin. *Free Radic. Res.* 27:311-323.

Van der Meer, P., Lipsic, E., Henning, R. H., Boddeus, K., van der Velden, J., Voors, A. A., van Veldhuisen, D. J., van Gilst, W. H., Schoemaker, R. G. (2005) Erythropoietin induces neovascularization and improves cardiac function in rats with heart failure after myocardial infarction. *J. Am. Coll. Cardiol.* 46:125-133

Van der Meer, P., Voors, A. A., Lipsic, E., van Gilst, W. H., van Veldhuisen, D. J. (2004) Erythropoietin in cardiovascular diseases. *Eur. Heart J.* 25: 285-291

Velly, L., Pellegrini, L., Guillet, B., Bruder, N., Pisano, P. (2010) Erythropoietin 2nd cerebral protection after acute injuries: a double-edged sword? *Pharmacol. Ther.* 128:445-459

Verdier, F., Walrafen, P., Hubert, N., Chretien, S., Gisselbrecht, S., Lacombe, C., Mayeux, P. (2000) Proteasomes regulate the duration of erythropoietin receptor activation by controlling down-regulation of cell surface receptors. *J. Biol. Chem.* 275:18375-18381.

Wang, F. F., Kung, C. K., Goldwasser, E. (1985) Some chemical properties of human erythropoietin. *Endocrinology* 116:2286-2292

Wang, L., Harris, T. E., Roth, R. A., Lawrence, J. C., Jr. (2007) PRAS40 regulates mTORC1 kinase activity by functioning as a direct inhibitor of substrate binding. *J. Biol. Chem.* 282:20036-20044

Wang, L., Zhang, Z., Zhang, R., Hafner, M. S., Wong, H. K., Jiao, Z., Chopp, M. (2004) Erythropoietin up-regulates SOCS2 in neuronal progenitor cells derived from SVZ of adult rat. *Neuroreport* 15:1225-1229

Wang, L., Zhang, Z. G., Zhang, R. L., Gregg, S. R., Hozeska-Solgot, A., LeTourneau, Y., Wang, Y., Chopp, M. (2006) Matrix metalloproteinase 2 (MMP2) and MMP9 secreted by erythropoietin-activated endothelial cells promote neural progenitor cell migration. *J. Neurosci.* 26:5996-6003

Warnecke, C., Zaborowska, Z., Kurreck, J., Erdmann, V. A., Frei, U., Wiesener, M., Eckardt, K. U. (2004) Differentiating the functional role of hypoxia-inducible factor (HIF)-1alpha and HIF-2alpha (EPAS-1) by the use of RNA interference: erythropoietin is a HIF-2alpha target gene in Hep3B and Kelly cells. *Faseb J.* 18:1462-1464

Wenker, S. D., Chamorro, M. E., Vota, D. M., Callero, M. A., Vittori, D. C., Nesse, A. B. (2010) Differential antiapoptotic effect of erythropoietin on undifferentiated and retinoic acid-differentiated SH-SY5Y cells. *J. Cell Biochem.* 110:151-161

Winearls, C. G., Oliver, D. O., Pippard, M. J., Reid, C., Downing, M. R., Cotes, P. M. (1986) Effect of human erythropoietin derived from recombinant DNA on the anaemia of patients maintained by chronic haemodialysis. *Lancet* 2:1175-1178

Witthuhn, B. A., Quelle, F. W., Silvennoinen, O., Yi, T., Tang, B., Miura, O., Ihle, J. N. (1993) JAK2 associates with the erythropoietin receptor and is tyrosine phosphorylated and activated following stimulation with erythropoietin. *Cell* 74:227-236.

Wright, G. L., Hanlon, P., Amin, K., Steenbergen, C., Murphy, E., Arcasoy, M. O. (2004) Erythropoietin receptor expression in adult rat cardiomyocytes is associated with an acute cardioprotective effect for recombinant erythropoietin during ischemia-reperfusion injury. *Faseb J.* 18:1031-1033

Wu, D. W., Stark, K. C., Dunnington, D., Dillon, S. B., Yi, T., Jones, C., Pelus, L. M. (2000) SH2-Containing protein tyrosine phosphatase-1 (SHP-1) association with Jak2 in UT-7/Epo cells. *Blood Cells Mol. Dis.* 26:15-24

Wu, Y., Shang, Y., Sun, S., Liang, H., Liu, R. (2007) Erythropoietin prevents PC12 cells from 1-methyl-4-phenylpyridinium ion-induced apoptosis via the Akt/GSK-3beta/caspase-3 mediated signaling pathway. *Apoptosis* 12: 1365-1375

Xue, Y. Q., Ma, B. F., Zhao, L. R., Tatom, J. B., Li, B., Jiang, L. X., Klein, R. L., Duan, W. M. (2010) AAV9-mediated erythropoietin gene delivery into the brain protects nigral dopaminergic neurons in a rat model of Parkinson's disease. *Gene Ther.* 17:83-94

Xue, Y. Q., Zhao, L. R., Guo, W. P., Duan, W. M. (2007) Intrastriatal administration of erythropoietin protects dopaminergic neurons and improves neurobehavioral outcome in a rat model of Parkinson's disease. *Neuroscience* 146:1245-1258

Yamaji, R., Okada, T., Moriya, M., Naito, M., Tsuruo, T., Miyatake, K., Nakano, Y. (1996) Brain capillary endothelial cells express two forms of erythropoietin receptor mRNA. *Eur. J. Biochem.* 239:494-500.

Yasuda, H., Shima, N., Nakagawa, N., Yamaguchi, K., Kinosaki, M., Mochizuki, S., Tomoyasu, A., Yano, K., Goto, M., Murakami, A., Tsuda, E., Morinaga, T., Higashio, K., Udagawa, N., Takahashi, N., Suda, T. (1998) Osteoclast differentiation factor is a ligand for osteoprotegerin/osteoclastogenesis-inhibitory factor and is identical to TRANCE/RANKL. *Proc. Natl. Acad. Sci. US* 95:3597-3602

Yu, F., Sugawara, T., Maier, C. M., Hsieh, L. B., Chan, P. H. (2005) Akt/Bad signaling and motor neuron survival after spinal cord injury. *Neurobiol. Dis.* 20:491-499

Zanjani, E. D., Poster, J., Burlington, H., Mann, L. I., Wasserman, L. R. (1977) Liver as the primary site of erythropoietin formation in the fetus. *J. Lab. Clin. Med.* 89:640-644

Zhang, D., Zhang, F., Zhang, Y., Gao, X., Li, C., Ma, W., Cao, K. (2007) Erythropoietin enhances the angiogenic potency of autologous bone marrow stromal cells in a rat model of myocardial infarction. *Cardiology* 108:228-236

Zhang, J., Li, Y., Cui, Y., Chen, J., Lu, M., Elias, S. B., Chopp, M. (2005) Erythropoietin treatment improves neurological functional recovery in EAE mice. *Brain Res.* 1034:34-39

Zhao, Y., Wagner, F., Frank, S. J., Kraft, A. S. (1995) The amino-terminal portion of the JAK2 protein kinase is necessary for binding and phosphorylation of the granulocyte-macrophage colony- stimulating factor receptor beta c chain. *J. Biol. Chem.* 270:13814-13818.

Zhong, L., Bradley, J., Schubert, W., Ahmed, E., Adamis, A. P., Shima, D. T., Robinson, G. S., Ng, Y. S. (2007) Erythropoietin promotes survival of retinal ganglion cells in DBA/2J glaucoma mice. *Invest. Ophthalmol. Vis. Sci.* 48:1212-1218

Zhu, X., Perazella, M. A. (2006) Nonhematologic complications of erythropoietin therapy. *Semin. Dial.* 19:279-284

Zoncu, R., Efeyan, A., Sabatini, D. M. (2011) mTOR: from growth signal integration to cancer, diabetes and ageing. *Nat. Rev. Mol. Cell Biol.* 12:21-35

Zou, T., Rao, J. N., Guo, X., Liu, L., Zhang, H. M., Strauch, E. D., Bass, B. L., Wang, J. Y. (2004) NF-kappaB-mediated IAP expression induces resistance of intestinal epithelial cells to apoptosis after polyamine depletion. *Am. J. Physiol. Cell Physiol.* 286:C1009-1018

In: Cardiovascular System
Editors: M. Oberfield and Th. Speiser

ISBN: 978-1-62948-308-5
© 2014 Nova Science Publishers, Inc.

Chapter 2

Cardiovascular Morbidities in Rheumatoid Arthritis: Effects of Exercise on Cardiac Autonomic Function

D. C. Janse van Rensburg[1]*, A. Jansen van Rensburg[1], C. C. Grant[1], J. A. Ker[2] and L. Fletcher[3]

[1]Section Sports Medicine, University of Pretoria, Hatfield, Pretoria, Gauteng, South Africa
[2]Department of Internal Medicine, University of Pretoria, Hatfield, Pretoria, Gauteng, South Africa
[3]Department of Statistics, University of Pretoria, Hatfield, Pretoria, Gauteng, South Africa

Abstract

Rheumatoid Arthritis (RA) is a chronic, inflammatory disease of unknown cause and primarily considered a disease of the joints. However, a variety of extra-articular manifestations including cardiovascular (CV) involvement are well recognized. There is a growing

---

* E-mail address: christa.jansevanrensburg@up.ac.za.

body of literature supporting the evidence for excess cardiovascular risk in patients with RA. Possible etiopathogenesis include conventional risk factors (hypertension, abnormal body mass index, smoking, etc.), accelerated atherosclerosis i.e., due to inflammation (measured by high-sensitivity C-reactive protein (CRP) and autonomic dysfunction (either by increased disrhythmogenic potential or by neuronal pathways modulating inflammation).

The autonomic nervous system is one of a variety of neuronal pathways implicated in modifying inflammation. Abnormal autonomic function is characterized by decreased heart rate variability (HRV).This may induce an increased disrhytmogenic potential. Exercise has been identified as one of the most important behavioural strategies for cardiovascular disease prevention and sedentary individuals (like RA sufferers) will benefit by even a small increase in physical activity. Many studies in non-RA groups demonstrated that exercise will improve autonomic function, as measured by HRV.

The aim of this chapter is to describe the cardiac involvement in RA and to discuss the data available on the effects of exercise in RA. This will be followed by a description of an exercise intervention and the cardiovascular effects reported in a group of South African female RA sufferers. The chapter will conclude with recommendations for future research.

List of Abbreviations

ANS	-	Autonomic Nervous System
BMI	-	Body Mass Index
CRP	-	C-reactive protein
CV	-	Cardiovascular
CVD	-	Cardiovascular Disease
HRV	-	Heart Rate Variability
MI	-	Myocardial Infarction
NSAID	-	Non-Steroidal Anti-Inflammatory Drug
PWV	-	Pulse Wave Velocity
RA	-	Rheumatoid Arthritis
SLE	-	Systemic Lupus Erythematosus

1. Introduction

RA is a chronic, systemic, inflammatory disease with articular- and extra-articular manifestations. Females are affected twice as common as males and approximately 1% of the world's population suffers from RA. [1-3] The joint disease is characterized by inflammation of the synovium in a symmetrical fashion. Any joint can be affected, large or small, but the small joints are mostly involved in early disease. [3, 4] Ultimately, inflammation and pannus formation (pathological proliferation of the synovium) leads to tissue destruction, including: cartilage, bone, ligaments, tendons and blood vessels. [5]. Rheumatoid arthritis leads to various physical impairments in those suffering from the disease. Inhibition of muscle contraction as a result of joint effusion, muscle atrophy secondary to decreased activity levels, loss of joint motion, and reduced aerobic capacity due to systemic disease account for the main reasons. [6, 7] Extra-articular disease imposes an additional burden on these patients with compromised health and almost any organ can be affected by RA. [3]

Morbidity and mortality are increased due to joint and systemic involvement. [8, 9] Myocardial infarctions (MI) and cerebrovascular incidents (as a result of accelerated cerebrovascular- and coronary artery atherosclerosis) top the list for increased mortality. [8, 10, 11] Meune et al., in their study on trends in cardiovascular mortality in patients with RA, concluded that reducing cardiovascular mortality should remain a major consideration in RA management. [11]

RA can affect the cardiac system in many ways and many of the cardiac involvement are only found at post-mortem. [12] All structures can be involved, e.g., the pericardium (pericarditis), myocardium (myocarditis) and the endocardium (endocardial inflammation, valvular disease). Some other recognized cardiovascular (CV) diseases include atherosclerosis, conduction defects, coronary arteritis and aortitis. [13]

Alamanos et al., in their research made the statement that people with RA die prematurely. [14] Meune et al., reported a 60% increase in risk of CV death in RA patients compared to the general population [11], while Aviña-Zubieta et al., after doing an observational meta-analysis reported that the increased mortality risk in RA patients are largely due to the higher rate of CV death. [15] There is thus a growing body of evidence that recognizes the excess CV risk in patients suffering from RA. [8, 16-18] Figure 1 illustrates the complex interactions between RA characteristics, CV risk factors and other determinants in developing CV disease.

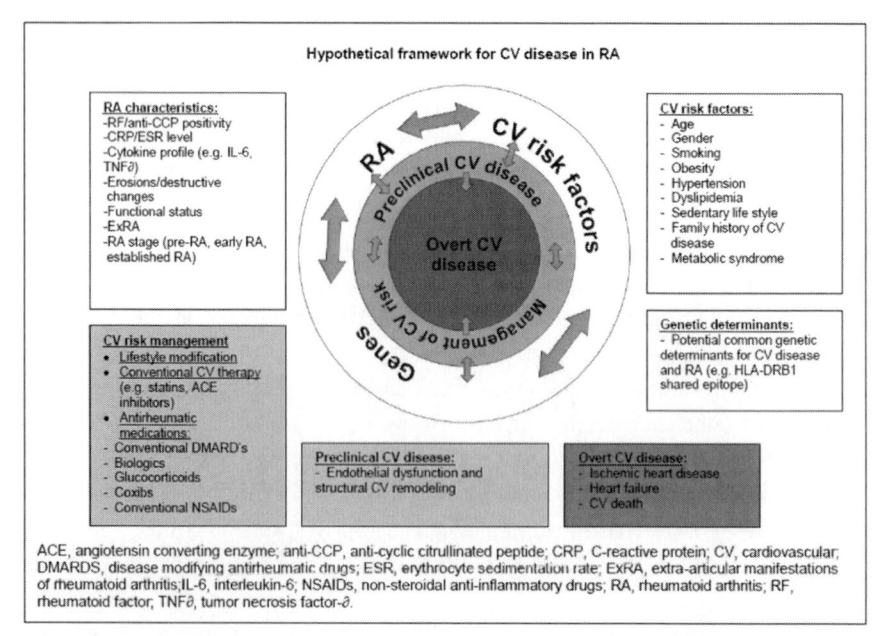

Figure 1. The complex interactions between RA characteristics, cardiovascular risk factors, genetic determinants and therapies on the development of preclinical and overt cardiovascular disease in RA [19].

Reproduced from Myasedova E, Gabriel SE, Cardiovascular disease in rheumatoid arthritis: a step forward. Current Opinion in Rheumatology 2010, 22:342-347. With permission from Wolters Kluwer Health.

Some of the hypotheses that have been generated to explain an increased risk of CV events are:

- The presence of conventional risk factors
- Accelerated atherosclerosis possibly induced by chronic inflammation
- Conduction disorders and arrhythmias

2. Cardiac Involvement

2.1. Conventional Cardiovascular Risk Factors

Gabriel in a recently published study evaluated the prevalence of traditional CV risk factors in RA as compared to non-RA subjects. The prevalence did not differ significantly at disease onset. Over the follow-up period when comparing RA and non-RA subjects for hypertension, high body mass index (BMI) or diabetes mellitus, there was also no significant difference. However, low BMI was significantly more common and hyperlipidaemia significantly less common comparing RA with non-RA subjects over time. [8] In Table 1 the prevalence of traditional risk factors are compared between RA (at disease onset) and non-RA patients:

Table 1. Prevalence of traditional cardiovascular risk factors at RA incidence in RA and non-RA patients [8]

	RA Patients	Non-RA Patients	
Cardiovascular risk factor	N%	N%	P Value
Cigarette smoking			<0.001
Never	285 (47)	341 (57)	
Former	148 (25)	118 (19)	
Current	170 (28)	144 (24)	
Hypertension	312 (52)	298 (49)	0.42
Dyslipidaemia	163 (49)	169 (52)	0.45
High BMI (>30 kg/m2)	71 (13)	68 (13)	0.98
Low BMI (<20 kg/m2)	73 (13)	63 (12)	0.50
Diabetes mellitus	44 (7)	41 (7)	0.74
Family cardiac history	287 (48)	284 (47)	0.86
Personal cardiac history	77 (13)	72 (12)	0.66
BMI, body mass index; RA, rheumatoid arthritis			

Reproduced from Annals of Rheumatic Disease, by SE Gabriel, Vol 69, page i62. Copyright notice 2013. With permission from BMJ Publishing Group Limited.

Gabriel then examined the impact of conventional risk factors on CV outcome, which was defined as a combined endpoint including heart failure, MI and CV death. Interestingly, a threefold increased risk of CV death was associated with a low BMI among RA patients. Lipids appeared to have a paradoxical effect, while the relative impact of the other risk factors (gender, smoking, personal- or family cardiac history, hypertension and diabetes mellitus) appeared to be significantly less in RA patients compared to non-RA patients (Figure 2).

The above findings were noted by other authors like Kitas and Avina-Zubieta, as well as Maradit-Kremers et al., who in their study concluded that "the risk of CV disease in RA precedes the American College of Rheumatology (ACR) criteria-based diagnosis of RA, and the risk cannot be explained by an increased incidence of traditional CV disease risk factors in RA patients". [15, 20, 21] Myasoedova commented that RA not only represents an important modifier of conventional CV risk factors, but also has a role to play as an independent risk factor. [19]

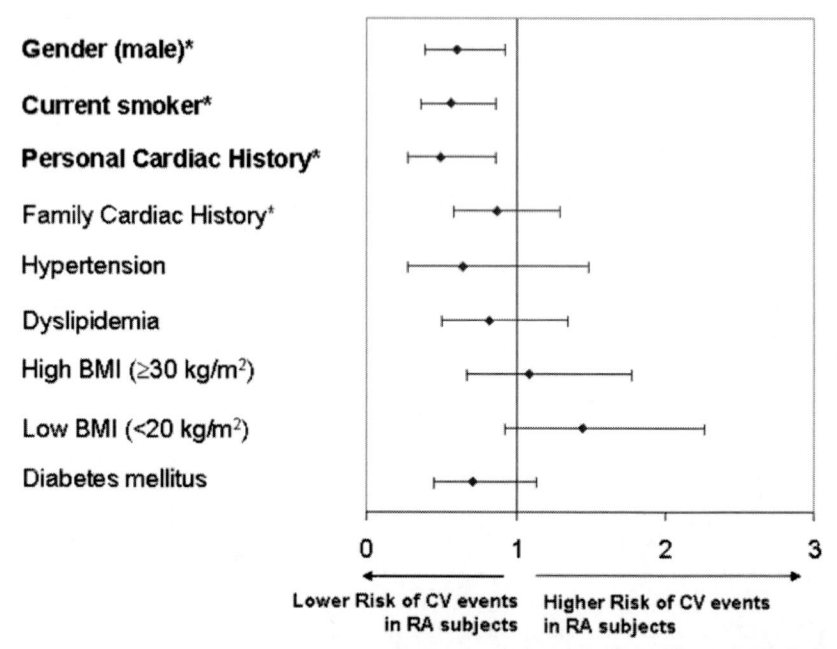

Figure 2. Relative impact of traditional CV risk factors on combined CV endpoint in RA and non-RA subjects [8].

Reproduced from Annals of Rheumatic Disease, by SE Gabriel, Vol 69, page i62. Copyright notice 2013. With permission from BMJ Publishing Group Limited.

Importantly the degree of target organ damage triggered by hypertension in RA patients remains fairly unidentified. In their study Panoulas VF et al., showed an increased occurrence of target organ damage in patients with RA who have no obvious CV or renal illness. [22] RA patients with target organ damage predominantly had either undiagnosed or uncontrolled hypertension, and target organ damage were mostly related to intravascular blood pressure oscillation, which highlights the value of early recognition and the management of high blood pressure in this patient group. [22]

Average blood pressure was proven to be the main independent determinant of arterial stiffness parameters, in both aortic augmentation index and carotid-radial pulse wave velocity (PWV), in RA patients. [23] Escalations in the average blood pressure also presented with an increase in arterial stiffness. The aortic augmentation index was influenced by RA as an autoimmune disease *per se*. Evaluating aortic augmentation index (indication of systemic arterial stiffness), carotid-radial PWV (indication of regional muscular vessel flexibility) and flow-mediated dilatation on brachial artery diameter (replicating endothelial function in the pre-atherosclerotic phase), may have a valuable diagnostic, prognostic, and therapeutic benefit. [23] PWV is an indicator of the stiffness of the arterial vessel, it replicates vascular dysfunction and is correlated to CV risk. Women with longstanding RA have a higher PWV in the upper limb arteries as compared to healthy controls and are comparable to patients with known traditional risk factors. [24]

2.2. Accelerated Atherosclerosis and Chronic Inflammation

There is compelling evidence that chronic inflammation has a pivotal role in the etiopathogenesis of atherosclerosis. [25] Several recent studies demonstrated the independent association of inflammatory indicators and RA towards an increased risk for CV disease. [8, 26-29] RA activity and severity, high CRP, erythrocyte sedimentation rate (ESR), rheumatoid factor (RF), anti-citrullinated peptide antibodies (ACPA) and HLA DRB1 gene are statistically significantly associated with increased risk of CV events. [27, 28, 30-33]

The 'SphygmoCor' pulse wave analysis (PWA) device was successfully used to assess arterial dysfunction in patients with RA. [24, 34-36], however the association between extra-articular manifestations and arterial dysfunction have not been assessed. PWA analysis using applanation tonometry at the radial artery, is a rapid non-invasive method for assessing central arterial function without the need for cardiac catheterisation, and can be used in a routine clinical practice. Assuming that the development of both atherosclerosis and extra-articular manifestations in patients with RA are related to the burden of systemic inflammation, then it might be predicted that patients who have demonstrated extra-articular manifestations could have a greater degree of arterial dysfunction than those without extra-articular manifestations. In a study by Crilly et al., arterial dysfunction increased as the number of extra-articular manifestations amplified. [37] Arterial dysfunction was however not related to the occurrence of rheumatoid nodules, Sjogren's syndrome or carpal tunnel syndrome. Crilly also found that severe extra-articular manifestations (including vasculitis, pericarditis and episcleritis) was related to increased arterial dysfunction, however the patient count was too small to validate that the finding was not coincidental. [37]

The Autonomic Nervous System (ANS) is one of a variety of neuronal pathways that have been implicated in modulating inflammation. [38] The "cholinergic anti-inflammatory pathway" is a well-studied mechanism where signals transmitted via the vagus nerve control the release of cytokines, reducing the production of pro-inflammatory cytokines by an α-7 nicotinic acetylcholine receptor (α7nAChR) dependent mechanism, and therefore ameliorating inflammatory disease. [39-41] Vlcek M, et al., evaluated the sympathoneural and adrenomedullary function of the ANS in young females with RA, compared to healthy controls. An orthostatic challenge which stimulates the sympathetic response in a different manner was included. [42] Epinephrine and norepinephrine plasma levels were monitored and the sympathoneural activity determined by HRV analysis. Similar responses in sympathoneural and adrenomedullary results were found and no difference in norepinephrine response to orthostatic challenge of RA patients compared to healthy controls. The normal heart rate and HRV observed indicates normal sympathetic response in young RA females. However several other authors showed reduced responses of the ANS. [43, 44] According to Vlcek the autonomic dysfunction to an orthostatic challenge in RA is a result of on-going inflammation on the disease development by dysregulation of immune functions. This might suggest that impairment of the sympathetic nervous system starts to develop at a later age. [42]

Recent studies have shown improved survival in animal models of inflammation by stimulation of the vagus nerve via electrical or pharmacological methods. [40, 45-47] Goldstein et al., in a prospective observational study found that RA patients had an increase in high mobility group box-1 (HMGB$_1$) – a pro-inflammatory cytokine – and a decrease in cholinergic anti-inflammatory pathway activity as measured by HRV. They postulated that it would be interesting to consider if subclinical CV disease is the result of increased inflammation secondary to decreased vagus nerve activity. [48] Vagus nerves have a vital role in regulating inflammatory reaction, via a primary neurotransmitter - acetylcholine (ACh) - an important facilitator of the 'cholinergic anti-inflammatory pathway'. [49] This neurotransmitter reacts with the nicotinic acetylcholine receptor (nAChR), specifically the α7 subunit (α7nAChR), as expressed by neurons, macrophages, primary fibroblast-like synoviocytes (FLS) and and other cells participating in the inflammatory response in the synovial tissue of RA patients. The stimulus of α7nAChR by ACh receptor withholds the release of pro-inflammatory cytokines. It was proposed that α7nAChR could be a marker for the management of RA. From this standpoint van Maanen et al., discuss the cholinergic anti-inflammatory pathway and its therapeutic potential in controlling arthritis activity. [49] Treatment with a specific α7nAChR agonists appears a favourable method for monitoring chronic inflammation. Alternatively, the divergent vagus nerve can be activated with a direct external electrical device, currently used in patients with neurological disorder. The inhibition of brain acetylcholinesterase could suppress chronic systemic inflammation in patients with RA, via the cholinergic anti-inflammatory pathway. [49] The presence of sympathetic nerve fibers in inflammatory contusions disappears shortly after the inflammation start. Owing to the immunosuppressive impact of sympathetic neurotransmitters at increased concentrations, the loss of sympathetic nerve fibers is compulsory in overcoming infection in inflamed and/or injured tissue. Fassold A et al., identified sympathetic nerve repellents in the synovial tissue of patients as possible contributing agents in RA. [50] On nerve terminals, repellent factors bind to neuropilin-2 and its co-receptor. However, soluble neuropilin-2 had no anti-repellent activity but triggered sympathetic nerve fiber aversion and arthritis. Increased shedding of neuropilin-2 is most probably an adverse sign in RA. It remains an open question whether or not the inhibition of neuropilin-2 shedding could mitigate the course of arthritis. Sympathetic nerve fibers and their steering control elements play a delicate role in the context of RA, osteoarthritis, and experimental arthritis. [50] In order to assess the hypothetical effect of systemic inflammation on HRV and ventricular repolarization (QT interval) in chronic inflammatory arthritis patients, a potential connection between HRV, QT interval and CRP was analysed. In patients with chronic inflammatory arthritis, the main conclusions Lazzerini et al., found was the following: [51]

(i) the degree of systemic inflammation, determined by CRP, is reversely related to HRV, and directly to QT duration;
(ii) patients that had high CRP levels presented both significant reduction in HRV and an extension of QT in respect to patients with a normal CRP value;
(iii) a parallel, although less noticeable degree of HRV reduction and QT extension was found in patients with RA when compared to patients with Spondyloarthritis and healthy controls.

The data provides confirmation of a relationship between systemic inflammation and the arrhythmic risk in patients with chronic inflammatory arthritis. [51]

2.3. Conduction Disorders and Arrhythmias

Conduction disturbances arise through impaired conduction or abnormalities of intrinsic automaticity. [52] Left atrial mechanical function is a key determining factor of left ventricular filling, particularly in patients with final-stage systolic and/or diastolic ventricular dysfunction, left ventricular hypertrophy, and decreased left ventricular enlargement capacity. A study by Acar et al., on RA patients showed substantially impaired left atrial mechanical functions. [53] They speculate that the decrease in the left atrial passive emptying action is linked to increased end-diastolic left ventricular pressure, and the raised left atrial active emptying capacity is related with a compensating action in left atrial contraction. A tissue Doppler imaging assessment revealed that intra- and interatrial electromechanical delays were significantly extended in RA patients. The interatrial electromechanical delay was also related to left atrial active emptying action and serum CRP levels. [53]

As the heart is richly innervated by efferent and afferent sympathetic and vagal fibers, it is highly susceptible to autonomic influences. [54] Zipes et al., had already in 1995 described the autonomic modulation of cardiac arrhythmias. Electrophysiological mechanisms underlying disrhythmogenesis are influenced by increased sympathetic and decreased vagal tone. [55, 56]

As reported in several non-rheumatic and rheumatic conditions, the ANS dysfunction is revealed by a variety of disorders that may occur in isolation or in various combinations and pertain to irregularity in blood pressure regulation, thermoregulation, gastrointestinal function, sweating, sexual function, sphincter control, ocular function and respiration amongst others. [57] Although the dysfunction of the ANS in RA patients has been well characterized and is related to high morbidity in diseases such as diabetes mellitus, its occurrence, symptoms, pathogenic development, management and prediction in RA patients remain mostly unknown. [57] Autonomic neuropathy may arise as a secondary concern of several diseases, however some patients lacking noticeable primary indicators show intense autonomic dysfunctions from an early stage of the disease. These idiopathic or key cases could be divided into groups of autonomic neuropathies. RA is one of the secondary autonomic neuropathies. [58]

Primary autonomic neuropathy, which typically influences both the cholinergic and adrenergic functions, is subdivided into autoimmune autonomic ganglionopathy (AAG), acute autonomic and sensory neuropathy (AASN) and acute autonomic sensory and motor neuropathy (AASMN), and grouped according to the presence or absence of sensory or motor dysfunctions. Typically, persons with an acute or sub-acute single stage clinical progression have been diagnosed with one of these kinds of neuropathy. The identification of the antiganglionic acetylcholine receptor (AChR) antibody defined the inclusion of immune mechanisms in idiopathic diseases, particularly in cases with true autonomic neuropathy. Being able to test for antibody presence has significantly unfolded the perception of autonomic neuropathy to include diseases with a chronic progressive trend that imitate true autonomic failure. Recently studies based on the AChR antibody have confirmed AAG as a remote nosological body within immune-mediated neuropathies. [58]

AAG and pure autonomic failure are both rare illnesses, and medical laboratory findings to distinguish AAG from pure autonomic failure have not been evaluated conclusively. Preliminary evidence was provided that these diseases could be discerned by way of postganglionic sympathetic, noradrenergic sensitivity. [59] Persons with any one of these conditions have symptoms of baroreflex-cardiovagal and baroreflex-sympathoneural failure. Both disorders are characteristic of low plasma levels of catecholamines for the duration of supine rest, however plasma levels of endogenous catechols, dihydroxyphenylalanine (DOPA), dihydroxyphenylacetic acid (DOPAC), and dihydroxyphenylglycol (DHPG), appear to be lower in pure autonomic failure than in AAG. This difference most likely reflects lower norepinephrine formation in PAF, due to dispersed sympathetic noradrenergic nerve interruption. Pure autonomic failure require cardiac sympathetic nerve disruption, while cardiac sympathetic neuroimaging by thoracic 6-[18F] fluorodopamine scanning signifies intact myocardial sympathetic sensitivity in AAG. [59]

AAG is an attained immune-mediated condition that leads to autonomic failure with diverse representation, principally in patients with lower antibody titration results. The disorder is presumably triggered by antibodies to the ganglionic nicotinic AChR causing severe orthostatic intolerance, syncope, constipation, gastroparesis, urinary retention, dry mouth, dry eyes, blurred vision and anhidrosis. Clinical findings by Gibbons & Freeman revealed an S-shaped association between a drop in blood pressure and antibody titration values. A decrease in antibody titers to ≤1 nmol/l seems to amend the appearance of autonomic dysfunction that may well be explained by the temporary clinical progress seen following a plasma exchange. [60] Abnormal cardiovascular function was also found to be more predominant when antibody levels were >1 nmol/L. The relation between cardiovascular function and antibody levels was also realised before and after immunomodulatory therapy. These results suggest that patients with high antibody titrations pose extensive dysautonomia whereas persons with lower antibody levels could develop into, or express more restricted appearances. [60]

Koopman et al., speculates that it is not clear if the dysregulation of the ANS is instigated by a raise in sympathetic nervous system activity, in the event of stress for example, with a subsequent decrease in vagus nerve activity, or whether it is vice versa. [61] It seems reasonable that the autonomic imbalance observed in RA patients is, in part, responsible for maintaining the inflammatory state.

Research by Majoie et al., demonstrates that vagus nerve stimulation caused a rebalancing of the immune system in 11 patients with refractory epilepsy, compared to a control group. [62] The result of vagus nerve stimulation on pro- and anti-inflammatory cytokines in peripheral blood, suggests that vagus nerve stimulation might be a favorable approach in the treatment of RA patients. Records attained from numerous *in vitro* and *in vivo* studies suggest that remedial agents targeting the parasympathetic nervous system via the cholinergic anti-inflammatory pathway, or targeting the sympathetic nervous system via adrenergic receptors could be an essential future treatment possibility in RA patients. [61, 62]

Using standardized methods (time domain analysis, frequency domain analysis and poincaré plot analysis) to determine HRV parameters, a study done on a female RA group by Janse van Rensburg, et al., in 2012, showed less variability (i.e., less healthy heart) in comparison to the healthy control group, for all three methods used. [63] Results showed higher resting heart rate and lower variability in their autonomic system (i.e., decreased HRV, probable autonomic impairment), as well as a poorer response to posture change, thereby indicating an increased risk for arrhythmias in RA patients, and a higher burden of morbidity. Thus, the evaluation of a possible increased disrhythmogenic potential might be critical in planning the long-term management of RA patients. With the time domain method the heart rate at any point in time or the intermissions between consecutive QRS progressions in a continuous ECG is registered, including the normal-to-normal QRS complex, and average heart rate. [63] In a study compiled by Jahan et al., it was confirmed that substantial enhanced resting pulse rate and diastolic blood pressure in RA patients, could be credited to the lower parasympathetic higher sympathetic motion consistent with the observations made by other researchers. A lower average RR interval (interval between consecutive QRS progressions) and higher average heart rate suggest a reduced vagal variation and directly link higher sympathetic and reduced parasympathetic activity. [64]

Thayer et al., reports on a meta-analysis of neuroimaging done on the association between HRV and regional cerebral blood flow. They identified numerous areas, among others the amygdala and the medial prefrontal cortex (mPFC), that are linked to responses of threat (insecurity) and safety which are also associated with HRV. The heart and brain are bi-directionally connected, consequently the afferent outflow from the one will affect the other. The vagus nerve forms a fundamental part of this system and HRV may offer evidence of how heart rate fluctuations, facilitated by cortical-subcortical pathways, integrate brainstem activity and autonomic responses in an individual. Their work supports the suggestion that HRV may control the level to which a mPFC-navigated 'fundamental integration' structure is linked with the cells in the brainstem that directly regulate the heart, and that HRV may control essential functions related to adaptability and health. [65]

3. Role of Exercise

RA patients are usually sedentary, with patients tending to limit physical activity due to the perceived danger of eliciting pain or damaging their joints. [66, 67] Although there is still no cure for RA, much can be done to manage the condition. High-grade systemic inflammation and its vascular and metabolic effects have received considerable attention. Despite compelling evidence that exercise can play a significant role in the physical and psychosocial health of the general population there were few studies found investigating exercise interventions in relation to CV disease in RA. [68] In a review on self-declared daily energy expenditure Mancuso et al., used the 'Paffenbarger Physical Activity and Exercise Index' [69], to quantify physical activity in patients with RA compared to healthy controls. [70] Their results disclosed that RA patients had a lesser amount of weekly total energy expenditure from physical activity compared to control patients. This was largely due to a reduced amount of walking and not because of less strenuous activities. The low activity level was most probably not due to physical limitations, but rather to reasons such as existing joint symptoms, and the mind-set of avoiding physical activity being afraid of further amplifying the already aggravated inflammation. Encouraging sensible and relatively safe physical activity, like walking, should be of high importance in the approach to reduce CV risk in rheumatoid arthritis. [70]

Studies on exercise intervention in RA patients used resistance training [66, 71-79], or aerobic training [5, 80-92], or a combination of strength and aerobic training. [7, 93-100] Strength training on its own seems to have a positive effect on functional ability [101-103] and muscular strength. [104] Cycling, followed by aquatics, aerobic dancing and walking/running are most frequently used as the mode of exercise in aerobic training for RA patients. [68] Although weight-bearing (and therefore possible joint damage) is minimized due to buoyancy [81], Hurkmans et al., found that water-based training only showed limited evidence for a positive effect on aerobic capacity and muscle strength contrary to land-based exercise which showed moderate evidence. [105]

No Randomised Control Trials based on walking as the main focus have been conducted [68], while studies focusing on aquatics suggest improvement of aerobic capacity [86, 106, 107], muscle strength [74, 87] and psychological status. [86] Studies on combination training showed positive influence on both cardiorespiratory fitness and muscle strength. [93, 108] Unfortunately training regimes, methodology and outcomes differ widely, making conclusions difficult. In a review done by Hurkmans et al., published in the Cochrane Library, they only included 8 studies because methodological criteria differed so much. [105]

In their study, Chang et al., demonstrated (i) that the BMI of female Taiwanese RA patients were noticeably lower than that of the overall population; (ii) there is a remarkable association between the physical/psychological-region and VO_{2peak} for female RA patients, and (iii) that there is a significant association between the physical/psychological /environment-region and functional aerobic impairment for female RA patients. The quality of life of patients with RA is determined by a multitude of related factors - including personal attitudes, social set-ups, and aerobic fitness. [109]

Metsios and his partners investigated the link between physical activity levels and CV disease risk profile in patients with RA. [110] Substantial variances in systolic blood pressure, cholesterol, low-density lipoprotein, homeostasis model assessment, type-I plasminogen activator inhibitor antigen, tissue-type plasminogen activator antigen, homocysteine, fibrinogen, apolipoprotein B and von Willebrand Factor with a consistent deterioration from the physically active, to the physically inactive group were found. Multivariate statistics of differences disclosed that physical activity levels were substantially related to the differences in all of the above variances after modifying age, weight, sex, smoking status, along with RA disease activity and severity. This descriptive research suggests that RA patients who are physically inactive have substantially worse CV disease risk profile compared to patients that are physically active. Benefits of increased physical activity to CV disease risk in RA patients still needs to be accurately assessed. [110] Metsios mentions that exercise has been identified as one of the most important behavioural strategies for CV disease prevention and that sedentary individuals (like RA sufferers) will benefit by just a slight increase in physical activity. [68, 111, 112]

Table 2. Recent studies of physical exercise and the risk of cardiovascular disease

Parameter studied	Outcome	Population studied (reference)
Self-reported physical activity (high versus low)	Increased total life expectancy (3.6 years) and CVD-free life expectancy (3.2 years)	Framingham Heart Study (USA) [114]
Self-reported physical activity (moderate versus low)	Increased total life expectancy (1.4 years) and CVD-free life expectancy (1.2 years)	Framingham Heart Study (USA) [114]
Sports participation at least 5 h/week versus 1–2 h/week	Reduced risk of CVD overall, CHD and ischemic stroke	Multicenter health screening survey (Japan) [115]
Walking at least 1 h/day versus 0.5–1 h/day	Reduced risk of CVD overall and CHD, trend for ischemic stroke (NS)	Multicenter health screening survey (Japan) [115]
Exercise less than 1 h/week versus at least 3.5 h/week	Increased risk of CHD, independent of obesity (BMI and WHR)	US Nurses' Health Study [116]
Self-reported physical activity (validated against aerobic test) – high versus medium/low/never	Reduced risk of death from CVD with high activity – independent of blood pressure level	Health screening survey (single county, Norway) [117]
CVD, cardiovascular disease; CHD, coronary heart disease; NS, nonsignificant; BMI, body mass index; WHR, waist–hip ratio.			

Reproduced from Turesson C and Matteson E.L. Cardiovascular risk factors, fitness and physical activity in rheumatic diseases. Curr Opin Rheumatol. 2007 Mar;19(2):190-6. With permission from Wolters Kluwer Health.

In a review by Turesson and Matteson, they focus on recent results of risk factors for CV disease in subjects with rheumatic diseases, and survey the role of physical activity in the prevention of cardiovascular disease. They found far-reaching indications from a variety of well conducted, community-based studies to indicate the beneficial effect of physical exercise on the risk of CV disease in the general population (Table 2). [113]

Patients with rheumatoid arthritis should be inspired to participate in a healthy lifestyle, comprising of regular physical exercise. [113] Up to now the main focus of exercise therapy has been to improve physical capacity and functional ability. [66] By tradition, RA patients were recommended to exercise only at a low intensity, since the fear of intensifying joint pain, inflammation, and destruction. Therefore, only isometric and range-of-motion exercises were believed to be safe. Over the last 20 years, increased attention was given to high-intensity, weight-bearing exercises that improves aerobic capacity and muscle strength. Munneke and De Jong reviewed 20 random clinical studies of various authors relating to the success of intensive weight-bearing exercise rehabilitation in patients with RA. [118] In >50% of the studies, a favourable result were presented regarding at least 1of the subsequent parameters: muscle strength, aerobic capacity, and joint mobility. Functional ability (activity of daily living) did not change in most studies. Notably in all studies, disease activity, expressed as erythrocyte sedimentation rate (ESR), and the extent of tender and/or swollen joints lessened or remained unaffected. In 35% of the studies, a substantial reduction in disease activity was found. In the short run, patients with RA are able to exercise intensely without an upturn in pain and joint inflammation. At the moment there are little data regarding the consequence of intense weight-bearing exercises implemented over an extended period of time (i.e., >1 year) on possible joint destruction. [118]

4. Exercise Intervention

The use of exercise as part of the management of RA has been widely debated. The concept of total bed-rest was the standard of care since the late 1800's. Only in 1948 the undesirable effects of prolonged bed-rest were described, and exercise then resumed its role as part of RA treatment and rehabilitation. [119]

According to the American College of Sports Medicine the primary objectives of exercise therapy in patients with RA are to:

- Preserve or restore range of motion (ROM) and flexibility around affected joints
- Increase muscle strength and endurance to build joint stability
- Increase aerobic capacity in order to enhance psychological state and decrease the risk of cardiovascular disease. [120]

A comprehensive exercise program for RA patients is said to include aerobic exercises at a moderate intensity for 3-5 days a week, isometric and/or isotonic strength training exercises 3 days a week and stretching exercise once daily. [121]

Previous studies in non-RA groups demonstrated that endurance exercise will improve HRV (i.e., cardiac health) [122-128], while strength training can have the opposite effect. [129] Many previous studies done on diseased populations to evaluate the effect of short-term exercise intervention on short-term HRV modification, assessed only supine variables. [130-139]

The HRV indicators are listed in Table 3 with an explanation of the efferent source of stimulation (sympathetic or parasympathetic branch of ANS). [140, 141]

Sandercock observed significant increases in the supine RR-interval, SDRR, LF(ln) and HF(ln) in a group of patients, who had coronary artery bypass grafting and angioplasty following myocardial infarction, after 8 weeks of cardiac rehabilitation. [130] Malfatto (1996) also showed significant increases for RR-interval, SDRR, RMSSD, pNN50 and HF but a decline in LF in patients who followed a training programme after MI. [136] On the other hand Oya et al., could not show any significant difference in HRV in MI patients after a 3 months training programme. [133] Figueroa observed a significant increase in LF and HF in a 16 week study in obese women with and without type 2 diabetes mellitus. [139] All the above mentioned studies (except Oya), thus showed increased vagal tone (HF, RMSSD, pNN50) after exercise intervention, but the LF variable seems to be difficult to interpret with changes in different directions in the various studies.

An exercise intervention study done by Janse van Rensburg, et al., in 2012 focused on the effect of cardiac autoimmune function in RA patients. [142] It was demonstrated that exercise intervention had a positive effect on autonomic function of RA patients, as measured by short-term HRV. Comparing the exercise group to the control group at baseline, the control group showed higher HRV. However, at completion of their study this changed in favour of the exercise group who then showed better HRV. These results are similar to that of Jurca et al., who after eight weeks of moderate exercise training in healthy females, showed improved vagal modulation of heart rate on 10 minute resting ECGs. [143]

Table 3. HRV techniques, HRV indicators and origins of variability

Time domain analysis	RR(s)	The mean of the intervals between successive QRS complexes, result of vagal and sympathetic influence on HRV.
	RRSD(s)	Standard deviation of intervals between successive QRS complexes, indicator of vagal and sympathetic influence on HRV (Overall HRV).
	RMSSD(ms)	Root mean square of the standard deviation between RR-intervals, indicator of vagal influence.
	pNN50(%)	The percentage of successive RR-interval differences larger than 50ms computed over the entire recording, indicator of vagal influence on HRV.
Poincarè plot analysis	SD1(ms)	Indicator of the standard deviation of the immediate RR variability due to parasympathetic efferent (vagal) influence on the sino-atrial node.
	SD2(ms)	Indicator of the standard deviation of the slow variability of the heart rate. It is accepted that this value is representative of the global variation in HRV.
Frequency domain analysis	LF(ms^2)	Indicator of sympathetic influence, but also including a parasympathetic component.
	HF(ms^2)	Indicator of only parasympathetic influence.
	LF/HF	Indicator of autonomic balance.
	LF(nu)	LF (normalised units) represent the relative power of the LF component in proportion to the total power minus the VLF component, i.e., LF/(total power-VLF).
	HF(nu)	The HF (normalised units) represent the relative power of the HF component in proportion to the total power minus the VLF component, i.e., HF/(total power-VLF)

LF   Low frequency.
HF   High frequency.
VLF   Very low frequency.

In Janse van Rensburg's study, only the RR-interval increased significantly in the supine position, while the other variables did not show significant changes in favour of the exercise group. [142] It is not clear why increased vagal tone was not demonstrated in the supine position in this analysis; however Iwasaki did a study where HF and RR-interval increased early in the training of young previously sedentary subjects, but after one year HF regressed towards initial values whereas RR-interval uniformly increased. They suggested that initial increases may be due to higher vagal modulation, while other factors such as heart geometry may play a role in further adaptation. [144]

In the RA group it was mainly the standing variables that were affected favourably in the exercise group in comparison to the control group. [142] Zoppini had similar results in a study on patients with type 2 diabetes mellitus where they showed significant changes in standing, but not supine variables after a six months exercise programme. [145]

The changes in the RA group reflected a greater effect on increased vagal rather than decreased sympathetic influence. [142] Buch in 2002 pointed out that patients may have a better survival advantage with enhanced vagal tone. Reasons offered were that greater vagal influence will: decrease heart rate and myocardial contractility (i.e., due to less workload and oxygen consumption); hinder sympathetic influence on the sinus node; and reduce the risk of ventricular disrhythmias. [146] Therefore, improving the vagal tone in RA patients may be an instrument to decrease their CV morbidity and mortality.

If the many possible factors contributing to the CV risk factor profile in RA patients is taken into account, there are many other factors that may well influence cardiac autoimmune function. De Meersman commented that "Ultimately, all of these CV diseases are associated with a common denominator, namely a perturbed autonomic balance. It is tempting, therefore, to hypothesize that preservation of cardiac autonomic function by lifestyle or interventions should be associated with a marked reduction in the risk of CV disease and death". [147] Exercise intervention appears to have an advantageous effect on cardiac autonomic function in RA patients as measured by short-term HRV. Especially vagal modulation seems to improve and this can lead to improved cardiac health in a patient group already suffering from impaired lifestyle due to joint pain and other complications following a diagnosis of RA.

Conclusion

RA patients have an increased risk of morbidity and mortality due to CV disease. Exercise has been identified as one of the most important behavioural strategies for CV disease prevention, and sedentary individuals (like RA sufferers) will benefit by just a slight increase in physical activity.

Study results by Janse van Rensburg, et al., in 2012 indicated that 12 weeks of exercise intervention had a positive effect on cardiac autonomic function as measured by short-term HRV, in females with RA. Several of the standing variables indicated improved vagal influence on the heart rate. [142] Exercise can thus potentially be used as an instrument to improve cardiac health in a patient group known for increased cardiac morbidity. However the influence of exercise on the traditional independent CV risk factors in RA still needs to be researched.

Future Research

Future research should focus on the long term effect of exercise on cardiac autonomic function, the effect of exercise on other CV risk factors, and the duration of the effect of exercise after it was terminated in patients with RA.

References

[1] A. M. Wolfe. *Bull. Rheum. Dis.* 19, 518 (1968).
[2] T. W. Huizinga. *Curr. Rheumatol. Rep.* 4, 195 (2002).
[3] J. R. O'Dell. In: W. J. Koopman, L. W. Moreland, editors. *Arthritis and Allied Conditions: Textbook of Rheumatology*. Lippincott, Williams & Wilkin, Philadelphia (2005)
[4] D. C. Nieman. *ACSM'S Health & Fitness Journal* 4, 20 (2000).
[5] L. Noreau, H. Martineau, L. Roy, M. Belzile. *Am. J. Phys. Med. Rehabil.* 74, 19 (1995).
[6] J. E. Hicks. *J. Musculoskelet. Med.* 17, 991 (2000).
[7] C. H. van den Ende, F. C Breedveld, S. le Cessie, B. A. Dijkmans, A. W. de Mug, J. M. Hazes. E *Ann. Rheum. Dis.* 59, 615 (2000).
[8] S. E. Gabriel. *Ann. Rheum. Dis.* 69, i61 (2010).
[9] C. Turesson, W. M. O'Fallon, C. S. Crowson, S. E. Gabriel, E. L. Matteson. *J. Rheumatol.* 29, 62 (2002).
[10] S. Wallberg-Jonsson, K. Caidahl, N. Klintland, G. Nyberg, S. Rantapaa-Dahlqvist. *Scand. J. Rheumatol.* 37, 1 (2008).

[11] C. Meune. E. Touze, L. Trinquart, Y. Allanore. *Rheumatology* 48, 1309 (2009).
[12] R. C. Jeffery. Medicine 38, 167 (2010).
[13] G. S. Firestein. In: G. S. Firestein, W. N. Kelley. *Kelley's textbook of rheumatology*. Saunders/Elsevier, Philadelphia (2009).
[14] Y. Alamanos, P. V. Voulgari, A. A. Drosos. *Semin. Arthritis. Rheum.* 36, 182 (2006).
[15] J. A. Avina-Zubieta, H. K. Choi, M. Sadatsafavi, M. Etminan, J. M. Esdaile, D. Lacaille. *Arthritis Rheum.* 59, 1690 (2008).
[16] M. T. Nurmohamed. *Autoimmun Rev* 8, 663 (2009).
[17] H. John, G. Kitas, T. Toms, N. Goodson. *Best Pract. Res. Clin Rheumatol.* 23, 71(2009)
[18] I. A. Ku, J. B. Imboden, P. Y. Hsue, P. Ganz. Circ. J. 73, 977, (2009).
[19] E. Myasoedova, S. E. Gabriel. *C. Curr. Opin. Rheumatol.* 22, 342 (2010).
[20] G. D. Kitas, S. E. Gabriel. *Ann. Rheum. Dis.* 70, 8 (2011).
[21] H. Maradit-Kremers, C. S. Crowson, P. J. Nicola, K. V. Ballman, V. L. Roger, S. J. Jacobsen, et al., Arthritis Rheum. 52, 402 (2005).
[22] V. F. Panoulas, T. E. Toms, G. S. Metsios, A. Stavropoulos-Kalinoglou, A. Kosovitsas, H. J. Milionis, et al., *Atherosclerosis* 209, 255 (2010).
[23] A. Cypiene, J. Dadoniene, R. Rugiene, L. Ryliškyte, M. Kovaite, Z Petrulioniene, et al., *Medicina (Kaunas)* 46, 522 (2010).
[24] H. Pieringer, S. Schumacher, U. Stuby, G. Biesenbach. Semin. Arthritis Rheum. 39, 163 (2009).
[25] R. Ross. *Am. Heart J.* 138, S419 (1999).
[26] A. H. Kao, M. C. Wasko, S. Krishnaswami, J. Wagner, D. Edmundowicz, P. Shaw, et al., *Am. J. Cardiol.* 102, 755 (2008).
[27] Y. H.Rho, C. P. Chung, A. Oeser, J. Solus, Y. Asanuma, T. Sokka T, et al., *Arthritis Rheum.* 61, 1580 (2009).
[28] K. P. Liang, H. M. Kremers, C. S. Crowson, M. R. Snyder, T. M. Therneau, V. L. Roger, et al.,. J *Rheumatol* . 36, 2462 (2009).
[29] S. A. Provan, K. Angel, S. Odegard, P. Mowinckel, D. Atar, T. K. Kvien. *Arthritis Res. Ther.* 10, R70 (2008).
[30] H. Maradit-Kremers, P. J. Nicola, C. S. Crowson, K. V. Ballman, S. J. Jacobsen, V. L. Roger , et al., *Ann. Rheum. Dis.* 66, 76 (2007).
[31] T. M. Farragher, N. J. Goodson, H. Naseem, A. J. Silman, W. Thomson, D. SymmonsD, et al., *Arthritis Rheum.* 58, 359 (2008).

[32] F. J. Lopez-Longo, D. Oliver-Minarro, I. de la Torre, E. Gonzalez-Diaz de Rabago, S. Sanchez-Ramon, M. Rodriguez-Mahou, et al., *Arthritis Rheum.* 61, 419 (2009).
[33] G. Tomasson, T. Aspelund, T. Jonsson, H. Valdimarsson, D. T. Felson, V. Gudnason. *Ann. Rheum. Dis.* 69, 1649 (2010).
[34] I> Avalos, C. P.Chung, A. Oeser, T. Gebretsadik, A. Shintani, D. Kurnik, et al., *J. Rheumatol.* 34, 2388 (2007).
[35] K. M. Mäki-Petäjä., A. D. Booth, F. C. Hall, S. M. L. Wallace, J. Brown, C. M. McEniery, et al., *J. Am. Coll. Cardiol.* 50, 852 (2007).
[36] H. Pieringer, U. Stuby, E. Pohanka, G. Biesenbach G. R*heumatol. Int.* 30, 1335 (2010).
[37] M. A. Crilly, V. Kumar, H. J. Clark, D. J. Williams, A. G. Macdonald. *Rheumatol. Int.* 32, 1761 (2012) .
[38] J. M. Waldburger, G. S. Firestein. *Curr. Rheumatol. Re.p* 12, 370, (2010).
[39] K. J. Tracey. *Nature.*420, 853 (2002).
[40] L. V. Borovikova, S. Ivanova, M. Zhang, H. Yang, G. J. Botchkina, L. R. Watkins, et al., *Nature.* 405, 458 (2000).
[41] T. R. Bernik, S. G. Friedman, M. Ochani, R. DiRaimo, S. Susarla, C. J. Czura, et al., *J. Vasc. Sugr.* 36, 1231(2002).
[42] M. Vlcek, J. Rovensky, G. Eisenhofer, Z. Radikova, A. Penesova, J. Kerlik, et al., *Cell. Mol. Neurobiol.* 32, 897 (2012).
[43] L. Stojanovich, B. Milovanovich, S. R. de Luka, D. Popovich-Kuzmanovich, V. Bisenich, B. Djukanovich, et al., *Lupus.* 16, 181, (2007).
[44] R. Geenen, G. L. Godaert, J. W. Jacobs, M. L. Peters, J. W. Bijlsma. *J. Rheumatol.* 23, 258 (1996) .
[45] T. R. Bernik, S. G. Friedman, M. Ochani, R. DiRaimo, L. Ulloa, H. Yang, et al., *J. Exp. Med.* 18, 781, (2002).
[46] H. Wang, M. Yu, M. Ochani, C. A. Amella, M. Tanovic, S. Susarla et al., *Nature* 421, 384 (2003).
[47] V. A. Pavlov, M. Ochani, L. H. Yang, M. Gallowitsch-Puerta, K. Ochani, X. Lin, et al., *Crit. Care Med.* 35, 1139 (2007).
[48] R. S. Goldstein, A. Bruchfeld, L Yang, A. R. Qureshi, M. Gallowitsch-Puerta, N. B. Patel, et al., *Mol. Med.* 13, 210 (2007).
[49] M. A. van Maanen, M. J. Vervoordeldonk, P. P. Tak. *T. Nat. Rev. Rheumatol.* 5, 229 (2009) .
[50] A. Fassold, W. Falk, S. Anders, T. Hirsch, V. M. Mirsky, R. H. Straub. *Arthritis Rheum* 10, 2892 (2009).

[51] P. E. Lazzerini, M. Acampa, P. L. Capecchi, M. Hammoud, S. Maffei, S. Bisogno, et al., *Eur. J. Intern. Med.* 24, 368 (2013).
[52] P. M. Seferovic, A. D. Ristic, R. Maksimovic, D. S. Simeunovic, G. G. Ristic, G. Radovanovic, et al., *Rheumatology (Oxford)* 45, iv39 (2006).
[53] G. Acar, M. Sayarlioglu, A. Akçay, A. Sökmen, G. Sökmen, S. Yalçintas, et al., *Turk. Kardiyol. Dern. Ars.* 37, 447 (2009).
[54] W. Wang, R. *Ma. Heart Fail. Rev.* 5, 57 (2000).
[55] G. F. Hutchins, M. A. Miller, D. P. Zipes. In: D. P. Zipes, J Jalife. *Cardiac electrophysiology : from cell to bedside.* Saunders/Elsevier. Philadelphia Saunders/Elsevier; (2009).
[56] K. A. Ellenbogen, B. S. Stambler, M. A. Wood. In: D. P. Zipes DP, J. Jalife J. *Cardiac electrophysiology : from cell to bedside.* Saunders/Elsevier, Philadelphia (2009)
[57] C. Ramos-Remus, S. Duran-Barragan, J. Castillo-Ortiz. *Clin. Rheumatol.* 31, 1 (2012).
[58] H. Koike, H. Watanabe, G. Sobue. J. Neurol. *Neurosurg. Psychiatry.* 84, 98 (2013).
[59] D. S. Goldstein, C. Holmes, R. Imrich. *Auton. Neurosci.* 146, 18 (2009).
[60] C. H. Gibbons, R. Freeman. *Auton. Neurosci.* 146, 8 (2009).
[61] F. A. Koopman, S. P. Stoof, R. H. Straub, M. A. Van Maanen, M. J. Vervoordeldonk, P. P. Tak . *Mol. Med.* 17, 937 (2011).
[62] H. J. M. Majoie, K. Rijkers, M. W. Berfelo, J. A. R. J. Hulsman, A. Myint, M. Schwarz, et al., *Neuroimmunomodulation* 18, 52 (2011).
[63] D. C. Janse van Rensburg, J. A. Ker, C. C. Grant, Fletcher L. *Int. J. Rheum. Dis.* 15, 419 (2012).
[64] K. Jahan, N. Begum, S. Ferdousi. *J. Bangladesh. Soc. Physiol.* 7, 78 (2012).
[65] J. F. Thayer, F. Ahs, M. Fredrikson, J. J. Sollers, T. D. Wager. *Neurosci. Biobehav. Rev.* 36, 747 (2012).
[66] C. Ekdahl, S. I. Andersson, U. Moritz, B. Svensson. *Scand. J. Rheumatol.* 19, 17 (1990).
[67] C. H. Stenstrom, M. A. Minor. *Arthritis Rheum.* 49, 428 (2003).
[68] G. S. Metsios, A. Stavropoulos-Kalinoglou, J. J. Veldhuijzen van Zanten, G. J. Treharne, V. FF. Panoulas, K. M. Douglas, et al., *Rheumatology (Oxford)* 47, 239 (2008).
[69] R. S. Paffenbarger, A. L.Wing, R. T. Hyde. *Am. J. Epidemiol.* 142, 889 (1995).
[70] C. A. Mancuso, M. Rincon, W. Sayles, S. A.Paget. *Arthritis Rheum.* 57, 672 (2007).

[71] A. Hakkinen, K. Hakkinen, P. Hannonen. *Scand. J. Rheumatol.* 23, 237 (1994).
[72] T. M. Hansen, G. Hansen, A. M. Langgaard, J. O. Rasmussen. *Scand. J. Rheumatol.* 22, 107 (1993).
[73] C. Ekdahl, R. Ekman, I. Petersson, B. Svensson. *Int. J. Clin. Pharmacol. Res.* 14, 65 (1994).
[74] C. H. Stenstrom, B. Lindell, E. Swanberg, P. Swanberg, K. Harms-Ringdahl, R. Nordemar. *Scand. J. Rheumatol.* 20, 358 (1991).
[75] L. M. Bearne, D. L. Scott, M. V. Hurley. *Rheumatology (Oxford)* 41, 157 (2002).
[76] M. Munneke, Z. de Jong, A. H. Zwinderman, H. K. Ronday, D. van Schaardenburg, B. A. Dijkmans, et al., *Arthritis Rheum.* 53, 410 (2005).
[77] S. M. Marcora, A. B. Lemmey, P. J. Maddison. *J. Rheumatol.* 32, 1031 (2005).
[78] Z. de Jong, M. Munneke, A. H. Zwinderman, H. M. Kroon, K. H. Ronday, W. F. Lems, et al., *Ann. Rheum. Dis.* 63, 1399 (2004).
[79] R. Nordemar. *Scand. J. Rheumatol.* 10, 25 (1981).
[80] K. Lyngberg, B. Danneskiold-Samsoe, O. Halskov. *Clin. Exp. Rheumatol.* 6, 253 (1988).
[81] A. Bilberg, M. Ahlmen, K. Mannerkorpi. *Rheumatology (Oxford)* 44, 502 (2005).
[82] T. M. Harkcom, R. M. Lampman, B. F. Banwell, C. W. Castor. *Arthritis Rheum.* 28, 32 (1985).
[83] L. Noreau, H. Moffet, M. Drolet, E. Parent. *Am. J. Phys. Med. Rehabil.* 76, 109 (1997).
[84] L. H. Daltroy, C. Robb-Nicholson, M. D. Iversen, E. A. Wright, M. H. Liang. *Br. J. Rheumatol.* 34, 1064 (1995).
[85] W. B. Karper, B. W. Evans. *Am. J. Phys. Med.* 65, 167 (1986).
[86] J. Hall, S. M. Skevington, P. J. Maddison, K. Chapman. *Arthritis Care Res.* 9, 206 (1996).
[87] S. Sanford-Smith, M. MacKay-Lyons, S. Nunes-Clement. *Physiotherapy Canada* 40 (1998).
[88] S. G. Perlman, K. J. Connell, A. Clark, M. S. Robinson, P. Conlon, M. Gecht M, et al., *Arthritis Care Res.* 3, 29 (1990).
[89] B. Baslund, K. Lyngberg, V. Andersen, J. Halkjaer Kristensen, M. Hansen, M. Klokker, et al., *J. Appl. Physiol.* 75, 1691 (1993).
[90] S. Melton-Rogers, G. Hunter, J. Walter, P. Harrison. *Phys. Ther.* 76, 1058, (1996).

[91] B. Danneskiold-Samsoe, K. Lyngberg, T. Risum, M. Telling. *Scand. J. Rehabil. Med.* 19, 319 (1987).
[92] M. A. Minor, J. E. Hewett. *Arthritis Care Res* 8, 146 (1995).
[93] C. H. van den Ende, J. M. Hazes, S.le Cessie, W. J. Mulder, D. G. Belfor, F. C. Breedveld, et al., *Ann. Rheum. Dis.* 55, 798 (1996).
[94] C. H. Stenstrom. *J. Rheumatol.* 21, 627 (1994).
[95] A. Hakkinen, A. Pakarinen, P. Hannonen, H. Kautiainen, K. Nyman, W. J. Kraemer, et al., *Clin. Exp. Rheumatol.* 23, 505 (2005).
[96] A. Hakkinen, P. Hannonen, K. Nyman, T. Lyyski, K. Hakkinen. *Arthritis Rheum.* 49, 789 (2003).
[97] R. Nordemar, U. Berg, B. Ekblom, L. Edstrom. *Scand. J. Rheumatol.* 5, 233 (1976).
[98] Z. de Jong, M. Munneke, W. F. Lems, A. H. Zwinderman, H. M. Kroon, E. K. Pauwels, et al., *Arthritis Rheum.* 50, 1066 (2004).
[99] G. R. Komatireddy, R. W. Leitch, K. Cella, G. Browning, M. Minor. *J. Rheumatol.* 24, 1531 (1997)
[100] A. Hakkinen, T. Sokka, A. Kotaniemi, P. Hannonen. *Arthritis Rheum.* 44, 315 (2001).
[101] A. Hakkinen, T. Sokka, A. Kotaniemi, H. Kautiainen, I. Jappinen, L. Laitinen, et al., *J. Rheumatol.* 26, 1257 (1999).
[102] Z. de Jong, M. Munneke, A. H. Zwinderman, H. M. Kroon, A. Jansen, K. H. Ronday, et al., *Arthritis Rheum.* 48, 2415 (2003).
[103] K. K. Lyngberg, M. Harreby, H. Bentzen, B. Frost, B. Danneskiold-Samsoe. *Arch. Phys. Med. Rehabil.* 75, 1189 (1994).
[104] A. Hakkinen, T. Sokka, H. Kautiainen, A. Kotaniemi, P. Hannonen. *Ann. Rheum. Dis.* 63, 910 (2004).
[105] E. Hurkmans, F. J. van der Giesen, T. P. Vliet Vlieland, J. Schoones, E. C. Van den Ende. *Cochrane Database Syst Rev* Oct 7;(4)(4):CD006853 (2009).
[106] M. A. Minor, J. E. Hewett, R. R. Webel, S. K. Anderson, D. R. Kay. *Arthritis Rheum.* 32, 1396 (1989).
[107] R. Suomi, D. Collier. *Arch. Phys. Med. Rehabil.* 84, 1589 (2003).
[108] American College of Rheumatology Subcommittee on Rheumatoid Arthritis, Guidelines. *Arthritis Rheum.* 46, 328 (2002).
[109] C. Chang, C. Chiu, S. Hung, S. Lee, C. Lee, C. Huang, et al., *Clin. Rheumatol.* 28, 685 (2009).
[110] G. S. Metsios, A. Stavropoulos-Kalinoglou, V. F. Panoulas, M. Wilson, A. M. Nevill, Y. Koutedakis, et al., *Eur. J. Cardiovasc. Prev. Rehabil.* 16, 188 (2009).

[111] B. D. Duscha, C. A. Slentz, J. L. Johnson, J. A. Houmard, D. R. Bensimhon, K. J. Knetzger, et al., *Chest* 128, 2788 (2005).
[112] G. F. Fletcher. *Cardiol. Clin.* 14, 85 (1996).
[113] C. Turesson, E. L. Matteson. *Curr. Opin. Rheumatol.* 19, 190 (2007).
[114] O. H. Franco, C. de Laet, A. Peeters, J. Jonker, J. Mackenbach, W. Nuselder. *Arch. Intern. Med.* 165, 2355 (2005).
[115] H. Noda, H. Iso, H. Toyoshima, C. Date, A. Yamamoto, S. Kikuchi, et al., *J. Am. Coll. Cardiol.* 46, 1761 (2005).
[116] T. Y. Li, J. S. Rana, J. E Manson, W. C. Willett, M. J. Stampfer, G. A. Colditz, et al., *Circulation* 113, 499 (2006).
[117] L. J. Vatten, T. I. L. Nilsen, J. Holmen. *J. Hypertens.* 24, 1939 (2006).
[118] M. Munneke, Z. de Jong. *Int. J. SportMed.* 1, 1 (2001).
[119] A. E. Kirsteins, F. Dietz, S. M. Hwang. *Am. J. Phys. Med. Rehabil.* 70, 136 (1991).
[120] L. Armstrong, G. J. Balady, M. J. Berry. *ACSM Guidelines for Exercise Testing and Prescription*. Lippincott, Williams and Wilkins, Philadelphia (2006).
[121] A. L. Millar. *Action Plan for Arthritis: Your guide to pain-free movement. Human Kinetics;* American College of Sports Medicine, Champaign, (2003).
[122] M. Buchheit, C. Gindre. *Am. J. Physiol. Heart Circ. Physiol.* 291, H451 (2006).
[123] A. E. Aubert, B. Seps, F. Beckers. *Sports Med.* 33, 889 (2003).
[124] K. M. Madden, W. C. Levy, J. K. Stratton. *Clin. Invest. Med.* 29, 20 (2006).
[125] J. V. Freeman, F. E. Dewey, D. M. Hadley, J. Myers, V. F. Froelicher. *Prog. Cardiovasc. Dis.* 48, 342 (2006).
[126] A. J. Bowman, R. H. Clayton, A. Murray, J. W. Reed, M. M. Subhan, G. A. Ford. *Eur. J. Clin. Invest.* 27, 443 (1997).
[127] J. B. Carter, E. W. Banister, A. P. Blaber. *Sports Med.* 33, 33 (2003).
[128] G. Raczak, L. Danilowicz-Szymanowicz, M. Kobuszewska-Chwirot, W. Ratkowski, M. Figura-Chmielewska, M. Szwoch. *Kardiol. Pol.* 64, 135 (2006).
[129] R. C. Melo, R. J. Quiterio, A. C. Takahashi, E. Silva, L. E. Martins, A. M. Catai. *Br. J. Sports Med.* 42, 59 (2008).
[130] G. R. Sandercock, R. Grocott-Mason, D. A. Brodie. *Clin. Auton. Res.* 17, 39 (2007).
[131] S. E. Selig, M. F. Carey, D. G. Menzies, J. Patterson, R. H. Geerling, A. D. Williams AD, et al., *J. Card. Fail.* 10, 21 (2004).

[132] M. W. Tsai, W. C. Chie, T. B. Kuo, M. F. Chen, J. P. Liu, T. T. Chen, et al., *Phys. Ther.* 86, 626 (2006).
[133] M. Oya, H. Itoh, K. Kato, K. Tanabe, M. Murayama. *Jpn. Circ. J.* 63, 843 (1999).
[134] M. Pietila, K. Malminiemi, R. Vesalainen, T. Jartti, M. Teras, K. Nagren, et al., *J. Nucl. Med.* 43, 773 (2002).
[135] D. Lucini, R. V. Milani, G. Costantino, C. J. Lavie, A. Porta, M. Pagani. *Am. Heart J.* 143, 977 (2002).
[136] G. Malfatto, M. Facchini, R. Bragato, G. Branzi, L. Sala, G. Leonetti. *Eur. Heart. J.* 17, 532 (1996).
[137] G. Malfatto, M. Facchini, L. Sala, G. Branzi, R. Bragato, G. Leonetti. *Am. J. Cardiol.* 81, 834 (1998).
[138] F. Iellamo, J. M. Legramante, M. Massaro, G. Raimondi, A. Galante. *Circulation* 102, 2588 (2000).
[139] A. Figueroa, T. Baynard, B. Fernhall, R. Carhart, J. A. Kanaley. *Eur. J. Appl. Physiol.* 100, 437 (2007).
[140] A. J. Camman, M. Malik, J. T. Bigger, G. Breithardt, S. Cerutti, R. J. Cohen, P. Cournel. *Circulation* 93, 1043, (1996).
[141] L. Mourot, M. Bouhaddi, S. Perrey, J. D. Rouillon, J. Regnard. *Eur. J. Appl. Physiol.* 91, 79 (2004).
[142] D. C. Janse van Rensburg, J. A. Ker, C. C. Grant, L. Fletcher. *Clin. Rheumatol.* 31, 1155 (2012).
[143] R. Jurca, T. S. Church, G. M. Morss, A. N. Jordan, C. P. Earnest. *Am. Heart J.* 147, e21 (2004).
[144] K. Iwasaki, R. Zhang, J. H. Zuckerman, B. D. Levine. *J. Appl. Physiol.* 95, 1575 (2003).
[145] G. Zoppini, V. Cacciatori, M. L. Gemma, P. Moghetti, G. Targher, C. Zamboni, et al., *Diabet. Med.* 24, 370 (2007).
[146] A. N. Buch, J. H. Coote, J. N. Townend. *Exp. Physiol.* 87, 423 (2002).
[147] R. E. De Meersman, P. K. Stein. *Biol. Psychol.* 74, 165 (2007).

In: Cardiovascular System
Editors: M. Oberfield and Th. Speiser

ISBN: 978-1-62948-308-5
© 2014 Nova Science Publishers, Inc.

Chapter 3

Heart Rate Variability (HRV) Assessment of Physical Training Effects on Autonomic Cardiac Control

C. C. Grant[1,*], D. C. Janse van Rensburg[1], P. Sandroni[2] and L. Fletcher[3]

[1]Section Sports Medicine, Faculty of Health Sciences, University of Pretoria, Pretoria, South Africa
[2]Mayo Clinic, Rochester, MN, US
[3]Department of Statistics, University of Pretoria, Pretoria, South Africa

Abstract

This Chapter reports the effects of a standardised, intensive physical training programme (energy expenditure: 8485 kJ/day) on autonomic cardiac control of a large group of healthy participants (N=154). It was hypothesized that results of exercise induced changes on the autonomic nervous system (ANS) are dependent on the body position and should be assessed not only in the resting position. Heart rate variability (HRV) recordings were made in the supine, rising and standing positions.

---

[*] Corresponding author: Dr. C. C. Grant, E-mail: rina.grant@up.ac.za.

Analytical techniques used were time domain, frequency domain and non-linear (Poincaré) analysis.

The results of this study, for the supine position, showed an increase in resting vagal control of the heart, and a general increase in HRV by exercise programs. It also showed, with the aid of deductive reasoning, that lower post-exercise heart rate may result, not only from the exercise-induced increase in vagal activity, but that a decrease in sympathetic control of the heart contribute to it. The exercise intervention increased both vagal and sympathetic variation during rising, without redistribution of the spectral frequency component. After the intervention, sympathetic activity was increased, not only during rising, but also during the standing period. When the influence of the exercise intervention on the orthostatic response was assessed as the difference between the stationary standing period and supine, the exercise-improved orthostatic response was indicated as a, predominantly, increase in sympathetic control. The work from this study thus showed that measurement of the influence of exercise on ANS functioning are dependent on the body position and assessments should be done, not only in the resting position, but also during standing and during an orthostatic stressor.

Introduction

Regular physical activity has many health benefits such as the prevention of, or decreasing in, the incidence of coronary heart disease, positive changes in cardiovascular functioning and beneficial metabolic, psychological and neurovegetative effects [1-3].

Exercise based clinical interventions are widely recommended to reduce morbidity and all-cause mortality [4, 5]. The protective influence of exercise on the heart to counter damaging cardiac events is believed to be the result of adjusted influences by the autonomic nervous system (ANS) on, for example, heart rate (HR) and heart rate variability (HRV). However, certain questions remain as to the effects of exercise on ANS control of the heart [6-8].

It is generally known that the initial aerobic training-induced effects on indices of HRV were heterogenic and controversial [9-11].

According to Hautala et al. [1] reasons for this heterogeneity in reports may lay in age, small sample size, the duration and also the intensity of the intervention. However, there is a consistent body of evidence that exercise increases resting vagal cardiac control, in healthy as well as patient groups [1, 12-15].

Although it is theorized that posture change and an orthostatic challenge may highlight ANS changes better than the resting supine position [16, 17], and that reduced ANS responsiveness to an excitatory stimulus is seen as the most common feature of patho-physiological states [18], exercise induced changes in HRV during standing and in response to an orthostatic stressor is less known.

In this Chapter the influence of a standardised, intensive physical training programme, in a controlled environment, on ANS cardiac control by means of HRV quantification, is reported. The exercise induced changes in overall HRV were measured in the supine, rising and standing positions as well as the adjustments in orthostatic response. Analytical techniques used were time domain, frequency domain and non-linear (Poincaré) analysis.

It was hypothesized that results of exercise induced changes on ANS are dependent on the body position and should be assessed not only in the resting position but also during standing and during an orthostatic stressor. It was also hypothesized that it is possible to better distinguish between exercise induced changes in vagal and sympathetic influence by taking measurements in different body positions.

Methods

Study Type and Study Population

This was a prospective twelve week exercise intervention study with a self-control design. The volunteers were between 18 and 22 years of age, consisted of 100 males and 83 females, and were of predominantly African ethnicity (African = 171; Mixed = 5; Caucasian = 5; Indian = 2). Mass and body mass index remained relatively constant over the study period as can be seen in Table1. None of the participants were professional athletes or high level sport participants. Exclusion criteria included refusal to freely give written informed consent; history of cardiovascular, hepatic, respiratory or renal impairment, as well as pulmonary, metabolic, and orthopaedic disease requiring medical attention; lung/ respiratory tract infection in the previous two weeks; medication that could influence cardiovascular control and psychological disorders.

All participants were subjected to the same standardised 24 hour routine (exercise, diet and sleep) for the duration of the twelve week exercise intervention.

The calculated average basal metabolic rate (BMR) for participants, taking weight, age and sex into account, was 6371 kJ/day. This, in addition to the energy expenditure of the training and exercise activities, resulted in a calculated average energy consumption of 8485 kJ/day, which can be classified as a medium to high intensity exercise program [19].

The study protocol was submitted and approved by the Ethics Committee of the University. All participants gave written informed consent before commencement of the intervention.

Data Sampling and HRV Quantification

Participants were instructed not to exercise or drink any alcohol or caffeine the 24 hours before measurements. They were allowed to eat a low protein breakfast (cereal with milk) on the morning of testing. POLAR RS800 heart rate monitors were used to obtain RR interval data sets (tachograms) from participants at the start (pre-intervention) and at the end (post-intervention) of the twelve week exercise period. After a 2 min stabilisation period in the supine position, ten minute tachograms were obtained for supine and 10 minute tachograms during standing upright, leaning with their backs against a wall, feet 30cm apart and 30cm from the wall.

Data sets were exported and artefacts in RR interval data were removed with standard Polar software programmes with a low filter power and a minimum beat protection zone of six beats per minute. The RR interval sets were analysed using HRV Analysis Software 1.1 for windows developed by the Biomedical Signal Analysis Group, Department of Applied Physics, University of Kuopio, Finland.

Smoothness priors for trend and Model Eye programme settings were used for detrending with an Alpha value of 500. The autoregressive model order value was 16 and the interpolation rate was 4 Hz. Standard time domain, frequency domain and non-linear (Poincaré analysis) techniques were implemented [20, 21].

The Poincarè analysis method was included due to its applicability to data that include non-linear phenomena [20] and also non-stationary data sets [22]. With this method SD1 and SD2, were determined. SD1 is an indicator of the standard deviation of the immediate, or short term, RR variability due to parasympathetic efferent (vagal) influence on the sino-atrial node. SD2 is an indicator of the standard deviation of the long-term or slow variability of the heart rate representing global variation [21].

Recommended time domain HRV indicators such as STDRR, RMSSD and pNN50 were determined and reported with RR interval and heart rate. Spectral components analysed with frequency domain analysis included high frequency (HF), 0.15 – 0.40 Hz, low frequency (LF), 0.04 – 0.15 Hz, and the LF/HF ratio. The indicators LF/HF, LFnu and HFnu were used as indicators of autonomic balance or relative power distribution between the sympathetic and parasympathetic branches of the ANS [20]. LFnu (normalised units) represent the relative power of the LF component in proportion to the total power minus the VLF component, i.e., LF / (total power-VLF). The HFnu (normalised units) represent the relative power of the HF component in proportion to the total power minus the VLF component, i.e., HF / (total power -VLF), while LF/HF is used to assess the fractional distribution of power [20].

A minimum tachogram length of 1 minute is essential to assess the high frequency (HF) components, and at least 2 minutes for the low frequency LF components during HRV analysis [20]. In the current study the non-stationary period during rising were analysed separately. One tachogram in supine position (directly before rising), one tachogram during rising (0 to 180s), one tachogram during standing (180 sec to 360s standing) and one tachogram during continued standing (360s to 540s standing) were used for HRV quantification.

The orthostatic response was quantified by the percentage difference (%Δ) between the HRV indicator values obtained during the first stabilised standing period (180-360s) and that obtained during the supine position (%Δ HRV indicator value = [standing – supine]/ supine x100). In addition, the percentage change was also calculated between the non- stationary rising-to-standing period HRV values (0-180s) and supine, as well as between the second stationary standing period (360-540s) and supine.

Statistical Analysis

The T-test is based on the assumption of normality, hence it is necessary to confirm that this assumption is met. In this study the chi-square goodness-of-fit test was used due to the relatively large sample size (rather than a test such as Kolmogorov-Smirnov which is usually used for smaller samples). The Chi-Square test was applied to all data sets (HR, RR, RRSTD, RMSSD, pNN50, SD1, SD2, LF Power (ms^2), HF Power (ms^2), HF Power (nu.), LF Power (nu.) and LF/HF to determine which indicator values were non-normally distributed.

From these, RMSSD, pNN50, SD2, LF Power (ms^2), HF Power (ms^2) showed P-values < 0.05 providing statistical evidence of significant differences from the normal distribution. This violates the assumption of normality of the T-Test. In such cases, two options are available; transformation of the data (using ln or square root) to obtain a more symmetrical distribution; or the use of non-parametric tests. As interpretation of transformed variables may be complicated, it was decided to use the Wilcoxon signed rank test (95% confidence level) to assess exercise intervention induced changes in the non-normal distributed data sets and the Matched T-Test for the rest. These tests was also used to determine if there was a difference in the % change (%Δ) in HRV indicator values in response to an orthostatic stressor as measured before and after the training period.

Results

The anthropometric characteristics of the group are shown in Table 1. As can be seen the mass, and therefore the BMI, remained relatively constant over the period. In Table 2 the HRV indicator values and standard deviations for the supine, rising and standing periods are depicted including the level of significance in differences found between pre-and post-intervention values. All HRV indicators, except the standing ANS balance indicators, showed significant exercise induced changes. All vagal and mixed origin HRV indicators (sympathetic and vagal) showed significant increased variability, while the supine ANS balance indicators, LF/HF and LFnu, showed significant decreases.

Table 1. Anthropometric characteristics of the study group: Mean and standard deviation

Characteristic	Males Pre-Intervention	Males Post-intervention	Females Pre-Intervention	Females Post-intervention
Height (cm)	171.36 (SD=5.86)	171.36 (SD=5.86)	159.26 (SD=5.49)	159.26 (SD=5.49)
Mass (kg)	61.78 (SD=6.89)	63.18 (SD=6.61)	60.22 (SD=8.99)	60.04 (SD=7.48)
Body Mass Index ($kg.m^2$)	21.43 (SD=2.16)	22.42 (SD=2.47)	23.40 (SD=3.04)	22.52 (SD=2.34)

SD= Standard Deviation.

Table 2. Comparison of average HRV indicator values as determined before and after the exercise intervention for the Supine, Rising and Standing periods. The significance of difference (Pre Δ vs. Post Δ) was determined by the Matched t-test and Wilcoxon signed-rank test depending on distribution of data

Indicator	Pre (SD)	Post (SD)	P-value	Pre (SD)	Post (SD)	P-value
	Supine			Rising (0-180s)		
HR(bpm)	72.58 (10.94)	61.38 (9.96)	<0.0001	89.28 (12.49)	80.12 (12.14)	<0.0001
RR(ms)	0.85 (0.13)	1.01 (0.16)	<0.0001	0.70 (0.11)	0.78 (0.13)	<0.0001
STDRR(ms)	0.05 (0.02)	0.07 (0.03)	<0.0001	0.05 (0.02)	0.06 (0.02)	<0.0001
RMSSD(ms)	57.35 (33.36)	83.95 (44.72)	<0.0001	33.2 (20.73)	47.1 (26.26)	<0.0001
pNN50(%)	34.55 (21.83)	58.45 (22.03)	<0.0001	9.4 (13.96)	14.9 (17.10)	0.0003
SD1(ms)	44.72 (23.74)	64.61 (31.58)	<0.0001	24 (14.79)	34.2 (18.70)	<0.0001
SD2(ms)	72.8 (36.95)	86.1 (47.15)	0.0020	108 (49.0)	130.6 (54.31)	<0.0001
LF(ms^2)	243 (396.9)	329.5 (873.2)	0.017	356 (373.8)	472.5 (501.4)	0.0001
HF(ms^2)	288.5 (391.3)	525.5 (729.8)	<0.0001	89 (172.9)	161 (225.3)	<0.0001
LF/HF	0.96 (3.13)	0.64 (10.13)	0.044	3.82 (17.50)	3.46 (12.34)	0.93
LFnu	46.45 (19.99)	38.2 (19.16)	0.0022	76.2 (19.03)	73.55 (20.86)	0.47
HFnu	50.1 (19.28)	58.95 (20.38)	0.0071	19.6 (18.60)	22.15 (17.23)	0.96
	Standing (180-360s)			Standing (360-540s)		
HR(bpm)	91.83 (11.69)	81.95 (12.40)	<0.0001	93.10 (12.31)	82.46 (13.62)	<0.0001
RR(ms)	0.67 (0.10)	0.75 (0.12)	<0.0001	0.66 (0.10)	0.75 (0.12)	<0.0001
STDRR(ms)	0.03 (0.01)	0.041 (0.02)	<0.0001	0.03 (0.02)	0.05 (0.02)	<0.0001
RMSSD(ms)	22.2 (15.49)	32 (29.23)	<0.0001	19.65 (16.53)	31.15 (23.44)	<0.0001

Table 2. (Continued)

Indicator	Pre (SD)	Post (SD)	P-value	Pre (SD)	Post (SD)	P-value
	standing (180-360s)			Standing (360-540s)		
pNN50(%)	2.6 (12.57)	8.95 (17.16)	<0.0001	1.95 (12.27)	9.85 (17.30)	<0.0001
SD1(ms)	18.46 (11.03)	27.28 (18.45)	<0.0001	17.43 (11.43)	26.95 (16.71)	<0.0001
SD2(ms)	52.9 (25.55)	76.55 (34.98)	<0.0001	49.85 (25.61)	75.65 (34.48)	<0.0001
LF(ms^2)	155 (254.8)	285.5 (401.1)	<0.0001	143.5 (227.0)	344.5 (510.3)	<0.0001
HF(ms^2)	35 (105.9)	77.5 (210.6)	<0.0001	32.5 (91.5)	70.0 (187.0)	0.0002
LF/HF	4.91 (24.07)	4.86 (29.70)	0.94	4.47 (20.67)	4.44 (29.49)	0.92
LFnu	80.3 (19.50)	79.75 (18.73)	0.67	80.50 (18.38)	80.00 (17.05)	0.34
HFnu	16.4 (18.15)	16.7 (17.06)	0.52	17.75 (16.66)	17.55 (16.73)	0.48

HR=heart rate; bpm=beats per minute; RR= RR interval; HF=high-frequency components; LF=low-frequency components; pNN50= percentage of intervals differing by >50 ms from preceding interval; RMSSD=root mean square of successive differences in RR intervals; STDRR=standard deviation of RR interval; SD1=standard deviation of short term variability; SD2=standard deviation of the long-term variability s: seconds; SD=Standard Deviation.

The percentage exercise induced changes (pre-intervention vs. post-intervention) in the supine position are shown in Figure 1. All indicators were significantly different (P<0.05) after the exercise intervention. It illustrates how variability in vagal and mixed origin indicators increased, while the ANS balance indicators LF/HF and LFnu decreased. Table 3 shows the exercise induced changes (Δ) in orthostatic response when the orthostatic response was calculated as a) the difference between indicator values obtained during rising (0-180s) and supine, b) the difference between values of the first period of stabilisation in the standing position (180-360s) and supine and c) the difference between values obtain during the second period of standing (360-540s) and supine.

Indicators of vagal influence (RMSSD, pNN50, SD1, HFms^2), showed a significant exercise induced decrease when the orthostatic response was calculated from the values during rising, i.e., [(0-180s) − supine]/supine x100.

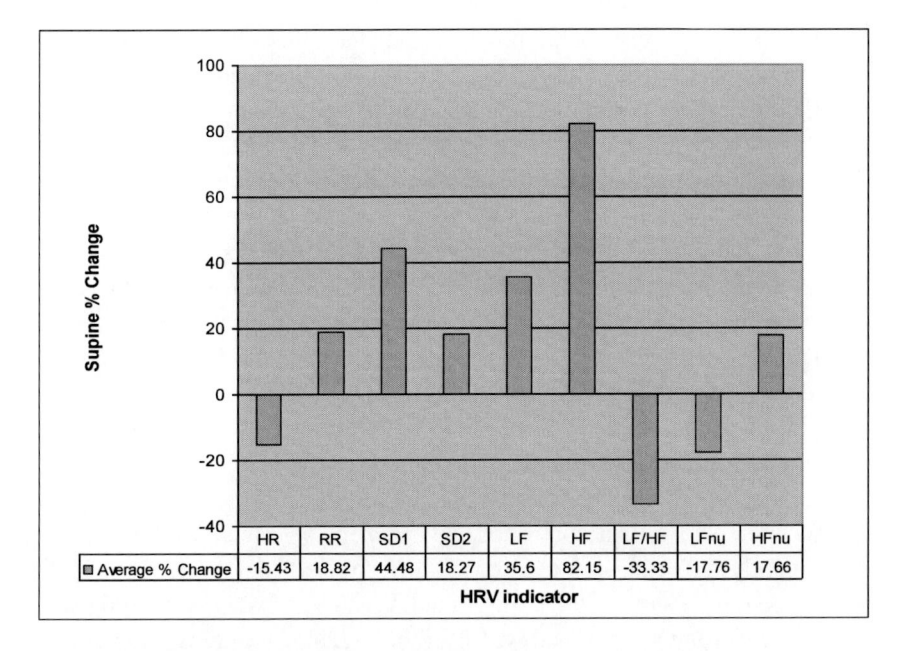

Figure 1. Percentage exercise induced changes on supine HRV indicators: [(Post exercise − pre-exercise)/pre-exercise] x 100.

HRV indicator	HR	RR	SD1	SD2	LF	HF	LF/HF	LFnu	HFnu
Average % Change	-15.43	18.82	44.48	18.27	35.6	82.15	-33.33	-17.76	17.66

However, when the response was calculated from either the first standing period i.e., [(180-360s) − supine]/supine x100 or, the second standing period, i.e., [(360-540s) − supine]/supine x100, no significant exercise induced changes was visible. In contrast, indicators of mixed origin (SD2, LFms^2) did not show significant exercise induced effects when the 0-180s period was used in the calculation, but showed significant increases when the 180-360s and 360-540s periods were used.

Discussion

Initially there were conflicting reports on the effects of exercise on the autonomic nervous system, but it is now generally accepted, at least for the supine position, that exercise can increase the vagal influence on the heart and thus the RR interval. However, from the positive, but relatively weak, association between the increase in RR interval and the increase in vagal activity [12], it is clear that the increase in the vagal regulatory input to the heart cannot be seen as the only contributor to the exercise-induced lowering of heart rate. In contrast to the now accepted fact that physical training can lead to an increase in the parasympathetic control of the heart, the effect on the sympathetic nervous system has not unequivocally been proved by HRV analysis.

As autonomic regulation of the heart is of paramount importance, not only in the supine position, but perhaps even more so during standing and in response to standing up from the supine position, it speaks for itself that the influence of exercise programs would perhaps be better assessed by measuring it in more than one position and in response to an orthostatic challenge. Although it is assumed that RR intervals sampled in the supine position is more reliable than during tilt or standing [12], Dietricha et al. [22] reported satisfactory reproducibility of these short–term, non-invasive measurements in the supine, as well as in the standing position.

The present study investigated the effect of a 12 week standardised exercise intervention in a controlled environment on a healthy young-adult, predominantly African, population. It investigated the influence of the intervention on the supine, the rising, standing HRV, as well as the orthostatic response. Recordings were analysed by time domain, frequency domain and Poincarè analyses. It was hypothesized that the influence of exercise on the vagal and sympathetic cardiac control, respectively, can be better assessed and understood by measurements in different positions.

The Influence of an Exercise Intervention on Heart Rate and RR Interval in the Supine and Standing Positions As Well As during an Orthostatic Stressor

In the present study the exercise intervention lead to a decreased HR and an increased RR interval in the supine, rising and standing positions (Table 2). HR was decreased by on average 15% in the supine position and 11% in the standing position, while the length of the RR intervals increased by 18% and 12%, respectively.

HR was significantly lower ($p<0.0001$) with RR and STDRR (standard deviation of RR interval) significantly higher ($p<0.0001$) during all four post-intervention tachogram periods (Table 2.).

The decrease in supine HR and increase in RR intervals are in line with previous publications, as reported in a 2005 meta-analysis of the effect of exercise on HRV in healthy participants [12] as well as that of a more recent review [14] on improvements in HRV with exercise therapy.

Table 3. The exercise induced changes (Δ) in orthostatic response determined during a) rising: (0-180s) rising HRV-supine HRV), b) (180-360s standing HRV-supine HRV) and c) (360-540s standing-supine). The significance of difference (Pre Δ vs. Post Δ) was determined by the Matched t-test and Wilcoxon signed-rank test depending on distribution of data

Indicator	Δ orthostatic response: % Change during rising = (0-180s rising-supine)			Δ orthostatic response: % Change during standing = (180-360s standing-supine)			Δ orthostatic response: % Change during continued standing = (360-540s standing-supine)		
	Pre	Post	P-value	Pre	Post	P-value	Pre	Post	P-value
ΔHR(bpm)	21.77	33.12	0.0001	26.32	36.75	0.0000	27.94	37.66	0.0001
ΔRR(ms)	-16.18	-22.86	0.0001	-20.07	-25.49	0.0000	-21.09	-25.72	0.0001
ΔSTDRR (ms)	2.53	-8.06	0.035	-26.46	-26.80	0.8582	-29.36	-25.93	0.5780
ΔRMSSD (ms)	-36.32	-46.79	0.0004	-57.05	-60.04	0.2334	-60.72	-60.79	0.5749
ΔpNN50(%)	-58.73	-70.41	0.0068	-88.18	-85.00	0.5311	-92.36	-80.82	0.0595
ΔSD1(ms)	-26.92	-39.82	0.0001	-49.86	-53.73	0.3194	-53.37	-54.00	0.4751
ΔSD2(ms)	55.15	46.53	0.8758	-28.02	10.76	0.0297	-30.77	-13.27	0.0234
ΔLF(ms^2)	67.12	54.52	0.8513	-23.66	-3.26	0.1178	-36.69	0.00	0.0395
ΔHF(ms^2)	-63.10	-72.79	0.0398	-84.08	-87.41	0.2686	-85.95	-85.98	0.4053
ΔLF/HF	269.49	480.00	0.0032	340	567.56	0.1304	331.73	535.09	0.0591
ΔLFnu	48.93	85.96	0.0232	157	131.57	0.0003	46.55	101.27	0.0004
ΔHFnu	-53.15	-63.88	0.0091	-53.4	-51.53	0.1085	-62.28	-70.24	0.1144

HR=heart rate; bpm=beats per minute; RR= RR interval; HF=high-frequency components; LF=low-frequency components; pNN50=percentage of intervals differing by >50 ms from preceding interval; RMSSD=root mean square of successive differences in RR intervals; STDRR=standard deviation of RR interval; SD1=standard deviation of short term variability; SD2=standard deviation of the long-term variability s: seconds; SD=Standard Deviation.

Several authors referred to the lowering of heart rate by exercise intervention as exercise-induced bradycardia [10, 12, 23, 24]. Textbook bradycardia is characterized by a heart rate below 60 beats per minute while normal resting rate is considered to be between 60 to 100 beats per minute [25]. Thus, although significant decreases in HR occurred in the present study, the twelve week, medium to high intensity intervention, did not result in bradycardia as the average supine heart rate of the participants were still above 60 beats per minute.

In addition to the lowering effect of the exercise intervention on the supine and on the standing heart rate, an effect was also seen on the heart rate during the orthostatic response. During rising from the supine position to the standing position the healthy heart will show an increase in rate. In the present study heart rate increased by 21.77% upon rising before the intervention, and by 33.12% post-intervention.

Before the exercise intervention a 16.18% decrease was found in the length of the RR-intervals upon rising (0-180s), with a post-intervention reduction of 22.86% (Table 3.). Thus a 7% lower increase in the length of the RR-interval upon rising after the 12 week exercise intervention than before the intervention. This is in agreement with Gilder et al. [6] who, in a cross-sectional study, showed a 6% higher decrease in RR-interval length in a low volume exercise group then in a high volume exercise group. It is said that these exercise induced changes measured in HR and RR interval during rising and standing, indicates increased responsiveness in the vagal reaction and sympathetic vasoconstrictor outflow upon stimulation of the baroreceptors [27].

STDRR is generally seen as an indicator of global variability. It is of interest, that both in this study and that of Gilder et al. [26]. STDRR over the period of rising, was 11% higher after the exercise intervention than before. In view of the relationship between HRV and health, this exercise induced increase in HRV, during the period generally marked by vagal withdrawal, once again illustrates the beneficial effect of exercise interventions on health.

Exercise Induced Changes in the Parasympathetic Autonomic (Vagal) Cardiac Control in the Supine and Standing Position Analysed by Time Domain, Frequency Domain and Poincarè Analyses

Results of this study (Table 2.) indicated that the average of all post-intervention indicators of pure parasympathetic (vagal) induced heart rate variation, as measured by RMSSD, pNN50, $HFms^2$ and SD1, were significantly higher ($p<0.0001$ to $p=0.0030$) than pre-intervention. This exercise-induced effect, as in the case for heart rate, was found for all 4 periods measured, i.e., in the supine position, during rising, as well as two standing periods.

A number of past studies reported conflicting results on the effect of exercise on the resting heart rate variability [28, 29].

Factors such as differences in study populations, exercise regimes and different analytical techniques (time domain, frequency domain and non-linear analysis), could have contributed to the differences [1, 30]. Nevertheless, at present the majority of cross sectional [1, 31-35], as well as longitudinal studies [1, 10, 36, 37], are in agreement that exercise can increase the vagal cardiac control. Unfortunately, the influence of exercise induced changes measured with short term HRV, are with some exeptions [38], mostly reported only for the supine position [12, 14].

Our results are thus in agreement with the current view on the effect of exercise on supine vagal control. In addition, it showed that exercise will also increase the average vagal influence during rising and standing. The results of the three HRV techniques were, although not in the magnitude of change, similar in the direction of change.

The Influence of an Exercise Intervention on the Sympathetic Autonomic HR Control in the Supine, Rising and Standing Position Analysed by Time Domain, Frequency Domain and Poincarè Analyses

Although it is often assumed that exercise can lower the sympathetic outflow to the heart, the HRV assessment of the sympathetic nervous system's response to exercise remains problematic. This is due to the fact that both sympathetic and parasympathetic influences are present in the LF heart rate oscillations [39]. The effect of exercise on sympathetic activity has also been assessed by measurement of muscle sympathetic nervous system activity (MSNA). However, these results also vary from increased, to decreased, to unchanged sympathetic activity [40, 41]. Results from the current study (Table 2) showed, not only significant increased variation in parasympathetic HRV indicators, but also in indicators of mixed origin (sympathetic activity + vagal activity), such as: STDRR, SD2 and LF(ms^2), over all four time periods. However, as shown in Figure 1., the exercise-induced increases in the average values of the mixed indicators (SD2:18.27%; LFms^2:35%) were, for the supine position, consistently lower than the exercise induced vagal increases (SD1:44%; HFms^2:82%). This did not apply to the rising and standing positions. The observation that the pure vagal influence increased more than the increase in the combination of the two branches is significant as it points towards an exercise-induced decrease in the supine sympathetic influence.

It is, however, not possible to state this empirically without examining the effects on the autonomic balance.

Results from the supine recordings on autonomic balance (Table 2) showed that the exercise intervention induced a significant shift towards increased parasympathetic influence, as seen in the pre- to post-intervention increase in HFnu (P=0.0071) and decreases in LF/HF (P=0.044) and LFnu (P=0.0022). The autonomic balance indicators for rising and standing did not show any exercise-induced changes.

The statistical significant supine values, especially LFnu, supported the notion of an exercise-induced decrease in the sympathetic influence in the supine position.

These findings of an exercise-induced increase in vagal and decrease in sympathetic activity during rest are, although in contrast to a number of other studies [23, 26, 42], in line with the conclusions in a review by Carter et al. [10] who reported endurance training to increase resting/supine HRV and parasympathetic activity while decreasing sympathetic activity.

When autonomic balance was taken into consideration, conclusions different from that of the supine was reached for the effects of the exercise intervention on the rising and standing position.

In this study, in agreement with Gilder et al. (2008) [26], no significant changes were found in the autonomic balance indicators during either the rising or the standing periods. The non-significance of the rising and standing exercise-induced changes in the LF/HF, LFnu en HFnu were thus probably due to an equivalent exercise-induced increase in average sympathetic outflow during rising and standing.

The findings of the present study of an increased parasympathetic and decreased sympathetic control in the supine position, are in line with the beneficial effects of a physical training program on the heart and with the lowering of resting heart rate.

As the weak association between the effect of exercise on the heart rate and that on the vagal influence suggests that other factors may play a role in the lowering of supine heart rate through exercise interventions, this exercise-induced reduction in the sympathetic outflow could very well make a considerable contribution [12].

In addition, an exercise-induced increase in sympathetic control during rising and standing would be in agreement with the normal homeostatic mechanisms involved in blood pressure regulation upon rising from the supine position, and with the beneficial effects of exercise to individuals prone to syncopy [43].

Influence of the Exercise Intervention on the Orthostatic Response Measured during 3 Different Tachogram Periods

HRV quantification of the response to rising from the supine to the standing position can give valuable insight into exercise induced ANS changes. Reduced ANS responsiveness to this type of excitatory stimulus is seen as the most common feature of patho physiological states [18]. It is said that postural changes, such as standing up, elicit sympathetic stimulation which, if attenuated, may be a marker of early sympathetic impairment [44]. However, it may also be an indication of exercise induced changes in the ANS. It is important to take cognisance of the fact that the orthostatic response can detect effects not visible in the supine position and that it can be a useful clinical tool to measure autonomic responsiveness, both in clinical medicine [45] and in exercise physiology [26].

Uniformity in the assessment of the ANS to an orthostatic response is problematic and periods and lengths of recording differ. The orthostatic response is generally seen as the difference between values obtained during the supine period and that obtained in response to the orthostatic stressor [18, 26, 43]. Complicating factors include uncertainties about the exact tachogram starting point during or after standing-up, the length of recording, which is critical due to the activation and normalisation of homeostatic mechanisms [46], and the importance of stationarity during HRV measurements [20]. The interpretation of when to record the values in response to the stressor differ. While the initial non-stationary period upon rising from the supine to the standing position is discarded by some authors [47, 48], others include this period [43, 46]. Even the length of this initial period, whether included or discarded, vary from 30 seconds [48], to two minutes [47], to 5 minutes [46], to 6 minutes [23].

In the present study, the vagal orthostatic response by the ANS was quantified by determining the % difference between supine vagal indicator values and that of rising/standing values at 0-180s, 180-360s and 360-540s, respectively. The difference between the pre-intervention and the post-intervention responses from supine to rising and standing are seen in Table 3. When the period during rising (standing 0-180s) was used for the calculation of the orthostatic response, highly significant exercise induced increases ($P<0.0001$ to $P=0.0398$) in vagal withdrawal (RMSSD, pNN50, SD1, HFms^2) were found from pre- to post-exercise intervention. The exercise intervention did not change the orthostatic response as reflected by the indicators of mixed origin (SD2: $P=0.8758$; LFms^2: $P=0.8513$).

It can thus be inferred that, for the indicators of mixed origin to stay the same, in the presence of a significantly larger vagal withdrawal, the sympathetic response must have increased during post-exercise rising. This was confirmed by the significant changes ($P<0.05$) in the values of the indicators of autonomic balance (LF/HF, LFnu and HFnu) in favour of increased sympathetic outflow, and the overall decrease in STDRR. These results are in agreement with the study by La Rovere et al. [49]. who reported, after 4 weeks exercise intervention, a significant higher resting-to-tilt increase in the LF component of HRV with a significant resting-to-tilt decrease in the HF component. The initial ANS orthostatic response to rising (0-180s), was thus significantly enhanced by the 12 week exercise intervention, both in terms of the vagal and sympathetic response.

The influence of the exercise intervention on the orthostatic response as calculated form the HRV values of the 180 to 360s period of standing minus the supine values was subsequently investigated. We have in a previous publication showed that HRV indicators already stabilized for the standing position during this period (180 to 360s after rising) [46]. No significant exercise- induced changes in pure vagal HR control (RMSSD, pNN50, SD1 and HFms^2 were found).

However, in the face of no exercise-induced change in vagal indicators, the increase in the SD2 indicator of non-linear rhythms and LFnu, showed a pre-post exercise induced increase in the sympathetic response.

In summary it can be said that the results discussed in this chapter are in agreement with the concept of a lowering of heart rate, an increase in resting vagal control of the heart and a general increase in HRV by exercise. The results further confirmed the assumption that a decrease in sympathetic control contributes to exercise-induced lowering of the resting heart rate. In addition, it was shown that both vagal and sympathetic control increased during rising without redistribution of spectral frequency components.

In contrast to the post-exercise increase in supine, rising and standing vagal activity, sympathetic activity, while lower at rest, was increased, not only during the period of rising, but also during the standing period. This, in the face of the post-exercise increase in vagal activity during standing, could be an expression of blood pressure maintenance in the standing position. When the effect of the exercise intervention on the orthostatic response was judged by using the values obtained over the non-stationary period (from supine-through-rising- to-standing) a significant stronger response was seen, both in terms of vagal withdrawal and sympathetic activity.

However, when the influence of the exercise intervention on the orthostatic response was assessed as the difference between the stationary standing period and supine, the exercise-improved orthostatic response was indicated as a predominantly sympathetic increase. It is thus clear that different results will be obtained on the influence of exercise, depending on the time of measurement relative to body position.

Conclusion

Results on the measurement of the influence of exercise on ANS functioning are dependent on the body position and assessments should be done, not only in the resting position, but also during standing and during an orthostatic stressor. It is possible to better distinguish between exercise-induced changes in vagal and sympathetic influence by taking measurements in different body positions and during orthostatic stress.

Future studies should compare, in patients with cardiovascular disorders, the value of investigations done only on supine recordings, to that done over three periods (supine, rising and standing). Based on the outcome of such studies, it will be possible to make recommendations for assessments in patients with cardiovascular disorders.

References

[1] A. J. Hautala, A. M. Kiviniemi and M. P. Tulppo. Review Individual responses to aerobic exercise: The role of the autonomic nervous system. *Neurosci. Biobehav. Rev.* 33, 107 (2009).

[2] R. J. Shepard, G. J. Balady. Exercise as cardiovascular therapy. *Circulation.* 99, 963 (1999).

[3] S. N. Blair, H. W. Kohl, R. S. Paffenbarger, D. G. Clark, K. Cooper, L. W. Gibbons. Physical fitness and all-cause mortality. *JAMA.* 262, 2395 (1989).

[4] O. R. N. Cortés, M. Heather and R. N. Arthur. Determinants of referral to cardiac rehabilitation programs in patients with coronary artery disease: A systematic review. *Am. Heart J.* 151(2), 249-256 (2006).

[5] S. Erbs, A. Linke and R. Hambrecht. Effects of exercise training on mortality in patients with coronary heart disease. References and further

reading may be available for this article. To view references and further reading you must purchase this article. *Coron. Artery Dis.* 17(3), 219-225 (2006).

[6] G. E. Billman. Cardiac autonomic neural remodelling and susceptibility to sudden cardiac death: effect of endurance exercise training. *Am. J. Physiol. Heart Circ. Physiol.* 297, H1171-H1193 (2009).

[7] F. S. Routledge, T. S. Campbell, J. A. McFetridge-Durdle, S. L. Bacon. Improvements in heart rate variability with exercise therapy. *Can. J. Cardiol.,* 26(6), 303–312 (2010).

[8] M. Mizuno, T. Kawada, A. Kamiya, T. Miyamoto, S. Shimizu, T. Shishido, S. A. Smith and M. Sugimachi. Exercise training augments the dynamic heart rate response to vagal but not sympathetic stimulation in rats. *Am. J. Physiol. Regul. Integr. Comp. Physiol.* 300, R969–R977 (2011).

[9] A. Aubert, B. Seps and F. Beckers. Heart rate variability in athletes. *Sports Med.* 33(12), 889-919 (2003).

[10] J. B. Carter, E. W. Banister and A. P. Blaber. Effect of endurance exercise on autonomic control of heart rate. *Sports Med.* 33(12), 889-919 (2003).

[11] K. Hottenrott, O. Hoos and H. D. Esperer. Heart rate variability and physical exercise: Current status. *Herz,* 31(6), 544-52 (2006).

[12] G. R. H. Sandercock, P. D. Bromley and D. A. Brodie. Effects of Exercise on Heart Rate Variability: Inferences from Meta-Analysis. *Med. Sci. Sports Exerc.* 37(3), 433–439 (2005).

[13] A. Borghi-Silva, A. R. Castello, R. P. Simo͂es, L. E. B. Martins, A. M. Catai and D. Costa. Aerobic exercise training improves autonomic nervous control in patients with COPD. *Respiratory Medicine.* 103, 1503-1510 (2009).

[14] F. S. Routledge, T. S. Campbell, J. A. McFetridge-Durdle and S. L. Bacon. Improvements in heart rate variability with exercise therapy. *Can. J. Cardiol.* 26(6), 303–312 (2010).

[15] S. T. Laing, T. J. Gluckman, K. M. Weinberg, M. K. Lahiri and J. Goldberger. Autonomic Effects of Exercise-Based Cardiac Rehabilitation. *J. Cardiopulm. Rehabil.* 31(2), 87–91 (2011).

[16] S. Guzzetti, E. Piccaluga, R. Casati, S. Cerutti, F. Lombardi, M. Pagani and A. Malliani. Sympathetic predominance in essential hypertension: a study employing spectral analysis of heart rate variability. *J. Hypertens.* 6(9), 711–17 (1988).

[17] F. Lombardi, A. Malliani, M. Pagani, et al. Heart rate variability and its sympatho-vagal modulation. *Cardiovasc. Res.* 32, 208–216 (1996).
[18] N. Montano, A. Porta, C. Cogliati, G. Costantino, E. Tobaldini, K. R. Casali and F Iellamo. Heart rate variability explored in the frequency domain: a tool to investigate the link between heart and behavior. *Neurosci. Biobehav. R.* 33(2),71-80 (2009).
[19] M. L. Foss and S. J. Keteyian. *Fox's Physiological Basis for Exercise and Sport*, McGraw-Hill, Dubuque, Iowa (1998).
[20] Task Force of the European Society of Cardiology and the North American Society of Pacing and Electrophysiology. *Heart rate variability: Standards of measurement, physiological interpretation and clinical use.* 93, 1043–1065(1996).
[21] L. Mourot, M. Bouhaddi, S. Perrey, J. D. Rouillon and J. Regnard. Quantitative Poincaré plot analysis of heart rate variability: effect of endurance training. *Eur. J. Appl. Physiol.* 91, 79-87 (2004).
[22] A. Dietricha, J. G. M. Rosmalenb, M. Althausa, A. M. Van Roonc, L. J. M. Mulderd, R. B. Mindera, A. J. Oldehinkelbe and H. Riese. Reproducibility of heart rate variability and baroreflex sensitivity measurements in children. *Biol. Psychol.* 85:71–78 (2010).
[23] F. S. Martinelli, M. P. T. Chacon-Mikhahil, L. E. B. Martins, E. C. Lima-Filho, R. Golfetti, M. A. Paschoal and L. Gallo-Junior. Heart rate variability in athletes and nonathletes at rest and during head-up tilt. *Braz. J. Med. Biol. Res.* 38(04), 639-647 (2005).
[24] R. L. Goldsmith, D. M. Bloomfield and E. T. Rosenwinkel. Exercise and autonomic function. *Coron. Artery Dis.* 11(2), 129-135 (2000).
[25] C. G. Blomqvist, B. Saltin. Cardiovascular Adaptations to Physical Training. *Ann. Rev. Physiol.* 45, 169-189 (1983).
[26] M. Gilder and R. Ramsbottom. Change in heart rate variability following orthostasis relates to volume of exercise in healthy woman. *Aut. Neurosci.* 143, 73–76 (2008).
[27] H. Kaufmann. Investigation of autonomic cardiovascular dysfunction. In: Korczyn, A. D., editor. Han*dbook of Autonomic Nervous System Dysfunction.* New York: Marcel Dekker Inc, 1995. pp. 427–68.
[28] S. H. Boutcher and P. Stein. Association between heart rate variability and training response in sedentary middle-aged men. *Eur. J. Appl. Physiol. Occup. Physiol.* 70, 75–80 (1995).
[29] B. C. Maciel, L. Gallo Junior, J. A. Marin Neto, E. C. Lima Filho, J. Terra Filho, J. C. Manco. Parasympathetic contribution to bradycardia

induced by endurance training in man. *Cardiovasc. Res.* 19, 642–648 (1985).

[30] G. R. H. Sandercock and D. A. Brodie. The use of heart rate variability measures to assess autonomic control during exercise. *Scand. J. Sci. Sports* 16, 302-313 (2006).

[31] R. L. Goldsmith, J. T. Bigger Jr, D. M. Bloomfield, R. C. Steinman. Physical fitness as a determinant of vagal modulation. *Med. Sci. Sports Exerc.* 29, 812–817 (1997).

[32] Ueno, L. M., Hamada, T., Moritani, T., et al. Cardiac autonomic nervous activities and cardiorespiratory fitness in older men. *A Biol. Sci. Med. Sci.* 57, M605–M610 (2002).

[33] M. Buchheit and C. Gindre. Cardiac parasympathetic regulation: respective associations with cardiorespiratory fitness and training load. *Am. J. Physiol. Heart Circ. Physiol.* 291, H451–H458 (2006).

[34] K. P. Davy, N. L. Miniclier, J. A. Taylor, E. T. Stevenson, D. R. Seals et al. Elevated heart rate variability in physically active postmenopausal women: a cardioprotective effect? *Am. J. Physiol.* 271, H455–H460 (1996).

[35] K. L. Rennie, H. Hemingway, M. Kumari, E. Brunner, M. Malik, M. Marmot, et al. Effects of moderate and vigorous physical activity on heart rate variability in a British study of civil servants. *Am. J. Epidemiol.* 158, 135–143 (2003).

[36] M. Al-Ani, S. M. Munir, M. White, J. Townend and J. H. Coote. Changes in R-R variability before and after endurance training measured by power spectral analysis and by the effect of isometric muscle contraction. *Eur. J. Appl. Physiol. Occup. Physiol.* 74, 397–403 (1996).

[37] E. L. Melanson and P. S. Freedson. The effect of endurance training on resting heart rate variability in sedentary adult males. *Eur. J. Appl. Physiol.* 85, 442–449 (2001).

[38] G. Zoppini, V. Cacciatori, M. L. Gemma, et al. Effect of moderate aerobic exercise on sympatho-vagal balance in type 2 diabetic patients. *Diabet. Med.* 24, 370-376 (2007).

[39] S. Akselrod, D. Gordon, F. A. Ubel, D. C. Shannon, A. C. Barger and R. J. Cohen. Power spectrum analysis of heart rate fluctuation: a quantitative probe of beat-to-beat cardiovascular control. *Science.* 213, 220 –222 (1981).

[40] B. Ekblom, A. Kilbom and J. Soltysiak. Physical training, bradycardia, and autonomic nervous system. *Scand. J. Clin. Lab. Invest.* 32, 251–256 (1973).

[41] S. F. Lewis, E. Nylander, P. Gad and N. H. Areskog. Non-autonomic component in bradycardia of endurance trained men at rest and during exercise. *Acta Physiol. Scand.* 109, 297–305 (1980).

[42] R. Jurca, T. S. Church, G. M. Morss, A. N. Jordan, C. P. Earnest. Eight weeks of moderate-intensity exercise training increases heart rate variability in sedentary postmenopausal women. *Am. Heart J.* 147, e21 (2004).

[43] M. R. Carnethon, D. Liao, G. W. Evans, W. E. Cascio, L. E. Chambless, W. D. Rosamond and G. Heiss. Does the Cardiac Autonomic Response to Postural Change Predict Incident Coronary Heart Disease and Mortality? *Am. J. Epidemiol.*, 155, 48–56 (2002).

[44] B. L. Mtinangi and R. Hainsworth. Increased orthostatic tolerance following moderate exercise training in patients with unexplained syncope. *Heart.* 80, 596-600 (1998).

[45] D. M. Bloomfield, M. D. E. S. Kaufman, T. Bigger jr., J. Fleiss, M. S. Rolnitzky and R. Steinman. Passive head-up tilt actively standing up produce similar overall changes in autonomic balance. *Am. Heart J.* 134, 316-320 (1997).

[46] C. C. Grant, D. C. Janse van Rensburg, N. Strydom and M. Viljoen. Importance of tachogram length and period of recording during non-invasive investigation of the autonomic nervous system. *Ann. Noninvasive Electrocardiol.* 16(2), 131–139 (2011).

[47] R. Perini, C. Orizio, S. Milesi, L. Biancardi, G. Baselli et al. Body position affects the powerspectrum of the heart rate variability during dynamic exercise. *European Journal of applied Physiology and occupational Physiology.* 66(3), 207-213(1993).

[48] K. Srinivasan, S. Sucharita and M. Vaz, Effects of standing on short term heart rate variability across age. *Clin. Physiol. Funct. Imaging.* 6 (22), 404-408.

[49] M. T. La Rovere, A. Mortara, G. Sandrone and F. Lombardi. Autonomic nervous system adaptations to short-term exercise training. *Chest.* 101, 299S-303S (1992).

In: Cardiovascular System
Editors: M. Oberfield and Th. Speiser

ISBN: 978-1-62948-308-5
© 2014 Nova Science Publishers, Inc.

Chapter 4

Autonomic Cardiovascular Control: Measurement and the Effects of Exercise

C. C. Grant[*,1], *D. C. Janse van Rensburg*[1], *P. Sandroni*[2] *and L. Fletcher*[3]

[1]Section Sports Medicine, Faculty of Health Sciences,
University of Pretoria, South Africa
[2]Mayo Clinic, Rochester, US
[3]Department of Statistics, University of Pretoria, South Africa

Abstract

Heart rate variability (HRV) analysis is a popular tool for the assessment of autonomic cardiac control. These measurements are increasingly employed in studies ranging from investigations of central autonomic regulation; to studies exploring the link between psychological processes and physiological functioning; to the indication of ANS activity in response to exercise, training and overtraining. Many publications elaborate on the effect of exercise on HRV and by implication on cardiac functioning. However, results on the effects of exercise on the autonomic control of the heart are often contradictory and incomplete in the normal population and in disease. In order to understand and employ the effects

---

[*] Corresponding Author: Dr CC Grant rina.grant@up.ac.za.

of exercise in patients with cardiovascular disorders it is of primary importance that agreement should be reached on the effects of exercise in the normal and healthy population.

In this chapter, a selection of older and more recent publications, investigating autonomic training effects as measured by cardiovascular variability indicators, are summarized. Reasons for heterogeneous results are identified and discussed. The chapter concludes with specific recommendations for future research.

Exercise is accepted to be of physical and psychological benefit for normal healthy individuals. However, it is also known to be of benefit in many types of physical and psychological disorders where it is associated with beneficial metabolic, psychological and neuro-vegetative effects [1].

Research has shown the benefits of exercise and training in controlling risk factors for coronary artery disease and in decreasing its incidence. Exercise studies in cardiac and hypertension patients showed that exercise may result in positive changes in the cardiovascular functioning [2, 3, 4]. Population-based studies have shown regular physical activity to be inversely proportional to long-term cardiovascular mortality when controlled for the presence of other risk factors in both men and women [5, 6]. The risk of coronary artery disease in physically inactive individuals are said to be twice that of their active counterparts. Importantly, the relative risk for cardiovascular mortality in the least fit or least active compared to the most fit or active, approaches a factor of six [5].

Even though exercise is often beneficial in individuals with cardiovascular problems, it is also in this group where it can have the more serious negative consequences. It is, for instance, reported that acute myocardial infarction may be precipitated by exercise. Studies have shown the relative risk of myocardial infarction within 1 hour after strenuous physical exertion, in those at risk, to be two to six times greater than that of comparable individuals who are sedentary or less active during the same time [7, 8, 9]. It is also known that endurance training and the presence of arrhythmias are linked by the fact that the 'Athlete's heart' (a physiological adaptation to extreme training), is a risk factor for the development of atrial fibrillation. Athlete's heart is a well-known consequence of endurance sport practice with symptoms such as dilatation, hypertrophy and above average enhanced vagal tone, indicating autonomic nervous system dysregulation [10]. Heidbüchel hypothesized that long-lasting, competitive endurance activities may induce right ventricle structural changes, leading to 'acquired right ventricular dysplasia'- thus increasing the risk of ventricular arrhythmias and sudden death [11]. There are also reports of endurance athletes showing enhanced parasympathetic activity that may co-exists with cardiac sympathetic excitation, also implicating autonomic nervous system (ANS) dysregulation [12].

As indicated by the above, high intensity exercise programs might require changes in the cardiovascular and autonomic nervous system that are not necessarily beneficial to the person. This poses the problem of the identification and measuring of what is and what is not healthy behaviour. In 2003 Heidbüchel and co-workers asked the fundamental question: what is the reasonable limit for the practice of sport and exercise? [11]. Mont and Brugada indicated the same year that endurance training may have harmful consequences for the heart, but that this needs to be confirmed by case-control studies of non-selected populations [13].

Heart rate variability (HRV) assessment is a popular tool for the assessment of autonomic cardiac control. Many publications exist on the effect of exercise on HRV and by implication on cardiac functioning. As demonstrated in the rest of Section 1, results on the effects of exercise on the autonomic control of the heart are often contradictory and incomplete in the normal population and in disease. In order to understand and employ the effects of exercise in patients with cardio vascular disorders it is of primary importance that agreement should be reached on the effects of exercise in the normal healthy population.

Autonomic control of the heart by sympathetic and parasympathetic modulation, is amongst others, assessed by the variability of heart rate [14-20] and blood pressure [21, 22]. Different frequency peaks reflect specific physiological stimuli and it is possible to estimate the involvement of the autonomic nervous system (ANS) influence and balance on heart rate (HR) regulation [14, 23, 24]. With power spectral analysis of HR, two characteristic peaks between 0.04 Hz and 0.15 Hz (A) and between 0.15 Hz and 0.5 Hz (B) are used to quantify the autonomic balance in terms of the low-frequency (LF)/high-frequency (HF) ratio [14, 24, 19]. Peak A is found in the region of Mayer waves (0.1 Hz) and is situated in the so-called LF area. It appears to be linked to the combined activities of the sympathetic and parasympathetic branches of the ANS. Peak B is synchronous with respiration, reflects vagal activity, is situated in the so-called HF area and also gives an indication of respiratory sinus arrhythmia (RSA) [14, 19]. During measurement of systolic blood pressure variability (BPV) the LF peak corresponds to sympathetic activity, while the HF peak is determined by mechanical effects of respiration on intra-thoracic pressure and cardiac filling [21, 22]. The variability in blood pressure and the corresponding physiological stimuli are difficult to identify. Indications are that the very low frequencies (≤0.04 Hz) are influenced by vascular tone, endothelium factors and thermoregulation, while the LF peak (0.07 - 0.15 Hz) relates to sympathetic activity and represents vasomotor tone [22, 23]. Baro-receptor sensitivity (BRS) reflects mainly vagal modulation of the HR by the arterial baroreceptors and the magnitude of response in heart beat interval to a change in blood pressure (ms/mmHg) [24].

In addition to frequency domain analysis, the HRV can be quantified with normal descriptive statistics called time domain analysis and by the Poincaré Plot analysis, also called return maps. The latter being a diagram (scatter gram) in which the RR intervals of the tachograms are plotted as a function of the preceding intervals [16].

The effect of exercise on the ANS as measured by cardiovascular variability quantification (HRV and BPV) can be summarised in three categories: the response of the ANS measured during a bout of exercise, [25-34] directly after a bout of exercise [31, 32, 35-42] and the long-term effect of regular exercise on the ANS (Table 1.) [34, 42-77].

The publications listed below and in Table 1 are included to indicate the differences in results published for the same variability indicators and is not a comprehensive meta-analysis of published material on the topic. Increases, decreases and no differences are demonstrated with the aid of signs (↑, ↓, ↔).

The Response of the ANS Measured during about of Exercise

A review by Sandercock et al., on HRV measured during exercise showed that the interpretation of variability measurements is difficult because indicators reflecting sympathovagal interactions at rest do not behave as expected during exercise and that the increased respiratory effort has a confounding effect on HF bands [25]. They concluded that standard HRV analysis during exercise is not recommended but that non-linear analyses methods and the use of coarse grain spectral analysis has potential and should be investigated.

The effect of fatigue and exercise effort may also act as a confounding factors on HRV measurements. It can be expected that HRV measurements will differ when taken shortly after exercise commencement when compared with measurements taken after prolonged exercise.

Banach et al., also expressed doubt on the applicability of the HRV power-spectrum analysis, with its present interpretation, to assess the sympathovagal interaction during exercise [26]. However, other authors encouraged the use of HRV components at rest and during exercise as prognostic indicators, but called for the refinement of exercise measurements [27] Eryonucu et al., used HRV as an indicator of ANS activity before, during and after exercise in a comparative study [28]. Two other studies reported increased sympathetic influence (measured by LF and LF/HF) on autonomic cardiac control during graded exercise [29, 30], including increased, peripheral, vascular sympathetic activation at 30% of maximum exercise in the study by Saito and Nakamura [30]. These results were in direct conflict with studies indicating significant suppression of both SNS and PNS autonomic cardiac control during graded exercise measured by the LF and HF of the power spectrum of HRV [32, 31]. In 1991 Yamamoto et al., [33] reported decreased PNS activity (HF) and unchanged SNS activity (LF/HF) up to 100% of the predetermined ventilatory threshold (T_{vent}), with an abrupt increase in SNS activity (LF/HF) only at 100% T_{vent}. Perini and Veicsteinas [34] concluded that changes in HF and LF power and in LF/HF observed during exercise do not reflect the decrease in vagal activity and the activation of the sympathetic nervous system (SNS) at increasing loads; neither do fitness level, age and hypoxia have any influence. However, exercising at medium-high intensities in the supine position did produce measurable increased power in LF (combination of vagal and sympathetic influence).

The Response of the ANS Measured after about of Exercise

There is still no general agreement on the activity of the ANS as measured during recovery. Heffernan et al., reported that cardiovascular variability measured during recovery from a single bout of endurance exercise indicated that the total power of HRV did not alter compared with significantly reduced total power found after resistance exercise [35]. However, the LF/HF ratio was significantly increased after both resistance and endurance exercise, indicating increased SNS (LF) and/or decreased PNS (HF) influence [35]. This corresponds with results published by Terziotti et al., who found a reduced HF (vagal) component of HR and decreased BRS during 15 minutes of recovery [36]. Another study [37] also found suppressed vagal (HF) activities during 10 minutes of recovery after 100% of the individual ventilatory threshold compared with baseline values. Raczak et al., found no differences in HF and LF activities between pre- and post-exercise measurements, but increased BRS and overall HRV as measured by SDNN (standard deviation of all intervals) after exercise [38]. However, Kamath et al., [31] and Figueroa et al., [42] reported significant increased LF power during post-exercise recovery. This contrasts with findings by Arai et al., who reported significantly decreased HR power at all frequencies compared with baseline values in normal subjects [32]. Decreased BRS and HRV after exercise were also reported in other studies [39, 40]. Lucini et al., reported that ageing progressively reduces the cardiac autonomic excitatory response to light exercise [41].

Long-Term Effect of Regular Exercise on the ANS

Table 1 shows findings on the long-term effect of regular exercise on the ANS [34, 42-77]. Techniques used to estimate cardiovascular variability were mostly time domain and spectral analysis of HRV. BRS was quantified by means of sequence technique and the alpha index, spectral analysis of BRS and also BRS by means of the slope of the baroreflex sequences and transfer function gain.

Articles on the effect of a training program over a period of time also showed a wide range of results. One study reported no change in baseline baro-receptor sensitivity (BRS) and HRV values after a 16-week fitness programme [42], while another found increased BRS when comparing fitness levels [43]. Aubert et al., also found no evidence of significant changes in resting autonomic modulation of the sinus node after a low-volume, moderate-intensity 1-year exercise programme [44]. Comparing 11 young sedentary participants and 10 endurance-trained cyclists Martinelli et al., found no difference in power-spectral components of HRV at rest [45]. However, a lower HR and higher values for time domain HRV indicators were reported during rest and head-up tilt, concluding that resting bradycardia seems to be more related to changes in intrinsic mechanisms than to ANS control modifications. Sharma et al., found no statistically significant changes in autonomic cardiovascular control of adult men measured by HRV after a physical training programme of 15 days [46].

Table 1. Examples of the regular/ long term exercise induced ANS responses reported for the same HRV indicators

Ref	First author	Participants	Review, intervention or cross sectional study	Main Results
42	Figueroa	8 female obese patients with T2D 12 female obese patients without T2D	16 weeks training	Spectral analysis of HRV BRS via sequence technique ↔HRV and BRS: no baseline changes
43	Spierer	48 healthy subjects & HIV patients (38 males)	Cross-sectional design	Spectral analysis of HRV BRS via alpha index; ↑BRS increased, ↑HF ↓LF/HF
44	Verheyden	14 sedentary men 15 controls	Intervention 1 year training	Spectral analysis of HRV ↔LF, HF, LF/HF
45	Martinelli	11 sedentary men 10 cyclists	Cross-sectional design	Spectral analysis of HRV ↑SDNN ↔LF, HF: SNS/PNS↔
46	Sharma	25 healthy males	15 days exercise training	Time domain and spectral analysis of HRV ↔HRV indicators
47	Buchheit	55 healthy subjects	Cross-sectional design	Time domain and spectral analysis of HRV ↑HF, RMSSD, pNN50
48	Raczak	24 healthy subjects (22 males)	Longitudinal design Long term training	Time domain and spectral analysis of HRV, spectral analysis of BRS ↑SDNN, pNN50, RMSSD, ↑Total power and LF ↑BRS

Table 1. (Continued)

Ref	First author	Participants	Review, intervention or cross sectional study	Main Results
49	Okazaki	10 healthy sedentary seniors, 10 masters athletes, 11 sedentary young men	Longitudinal (12 months) & Cross-sectional design	Spectral analysis of HRV BRS via transfer function gain ↑SDRR, LF, HF ↑BRS
50	Melo	41 healthy males	Cross-sectional design	Time domain and spectral analysis of HRV ↑RMSSD ↓HR
51	Goldsmith	NA	Literature review	Review ↓SNS activity ↑PNS activity
52	Goldsmith	37 healthy subjects	Cross-sectional design	Spectral analysis of HRV ↑HF
53	Kiviniemi	17 healthy males	8 weeks training	Spectral analysis of HRV ↑HF
54	Cooke	11 healthy males	4 weeks training	Time domain analysis of HRV, BRS; ↑SDRR ↑BRS
55	Costes	21 COPD patients, 18 healthy subjects	8 weeks rehabilitation programme	BRS via the slope of the baroreflex sequences between systolic blood pressure changes ↑BRS
56	Monahan	133 healthy males	Cross sectional and 3 months intervention	BRS via linear regression between BP en RR intervals during a Valsalva maneuver ↑BRS

Ref	First author	Participants	Review, intervention or cross sectional study	Main Results
57	Carter	Healthy participants, effects of age, gender	Review	↓SNS activity ↑PNS activity
58	Iellamo.	7 healthy subjects	Longitudinal design, seasonal training	Spectral analysis of HRV BRS via the sequences method 100% training load reverse effects: ↑LF,↓HF, BRS↓
59	Bowman	26 healthy subjects (16 males)	6 weeks aerobic training	BRS via the alpha index ↔BRS
60	Nagai	305 healthy subjects (167 males)	12 months exercise	Spectral analysis of HRV ↑LF, ↓HF
61	Pigozzi	26 female athletes	5 weeks training	Time domain and spectral analysis of HRV; ↔Time domain ↔ LF, HF (daytime)
62	Gulli	11 healthy females	6 months training	Spectral analysis of HRV and BPV ↑BRS ↑LF (RR), LF (SAP)
63	Goldsmith	16 healthy males	Cross-sectional design	Report conflicting results Spectral analysis of HRV ↑HF
64	Hautala	51 healthy men	8 weeks training	Baseline vagal (HF) influence determines effect of exercise training
65	Laoutaris	23 chronic heart failure patients	10 weeks training	↔HRV markers
66	Billman,	NA	Literature review	↑parasympathetic regulation, ↓sympathetic activity

Table 1. (Continued)

Ref	First author	Participants	Review, intervention or cross sectional study	Main Results
67	Borghi-Silva	40 COPD patients	6 week training	↑ sympathetic ↑ parasympathetic
68	Soares-Miranda	84 adults	Cross sectional	↑ vagal HRV
69	Sridhar	52 normotensive & 53 hypertensive diabetic patients	12 months training	↑ HRV
70	Cornelissen,	36 healthy subjects (17 males)	3x10 week crossover design	↓ HR ↓ ↔ sympathovagal balance
71	Kouidi	44 hemodialysis patients (20 controls)	1 year training	↑ SD of RR intervals ↑ MSSD ↑ pNN50
72	Knoepfli-Lenzin	57 healthy males	Longitudinal design	↑ supine heart rate variability
73	Routledge	NA	Literature review	↑ vagal tone ↓ sympathetic activity
74	Albinet	24 healthy subjects (11 males)	12 weeks training	↑ vagal-mediated HRV ↑ SDRR, ↑ RMSSD, ↑ HF power
75	Riesenberg	45 lung cancer patients	28 days rehabilitation	↑ HRV, ↑ RMSSD ↓ HR
76	Sato	20 coronary heart disease patients (13 males)	1 year Tai Chi conditioning	↑ BRS ↔ HRV
77	Kingsley	9 Fibromyalgia subjects, 15 health subjects (24 females)	12 weeks resistance exercise training	No significant effects of RET on HRV at rest or post exercise
78	Sandercock	Healthy subjects	Review	HF power ↑ RR interval ↑
79	Hautala	Clinical and sport	Review	↑ vagal tone ↓ Sympathetic inconsistent

Ref	First author	Participants	Review, intervention or cross sectional study	Main Results
80	Sandercock	28 patients (21 males)	8 weeks of cardiac rehabilitation	LFpower↑, HF↑, SDNN↑ RMSSD↑, LF:HF ratio↔
81	Laing	Patient coronary artery disease n=17	Intervention: Phase2 cardiac rehab	Recovery vagal influence↑ Resting RMSSD↔
82	Montano	Clinical and experimental populations	Review	↑Parasymp ↓Sympathetic
83	Billman	Clinical and experimental populations	Review	↑parasymp=enhance electrical stability
84	De Meerman	Aging population	Review	↑vagal tone in old age
85	Gademan	Clinical populations	Review	↓Sympathetic sympathoinhibitory effects in CHF
86	Montano	Clinical populations	Review	↑Parasymp ↓Sympathetic

Ref: Reference number, LF: Low frequency, HF: High frequency, SDNN: Standard deviation of all intervals, Ptot: Total frequency power, pNN50: Percentage of successive interval differences greater than 50ms, SNS: Sympathetic nervous system, PNS: Parasympathetic nervous system, SAP: Systolic arterial pressure, ↑:increase, ↓:decrease, ↔:no changes in variability indicators.

Perini and Veicsteinas [34] reported no influence of factors such as age and fitness level, while Bucheit and Gindre [47] showed that modifications in autonomic activities induced by training are visible in HRV power spectra at rest. Rackzak et al., [48] reported parasympathetic nervous system (PNS) dominance by measuring HRV and increased BRS after long-term exercise training. Another study reported increased HRV and BRS in Masters Athletes compared with decreased values for sedentary seniors [49]. Several other studies also concluded that regular physical activity increases vagal influence on the HR and BRS, while the sympathetic tone may be decreased [50-59]. However, Iellamo et al., [58] found a reversal of these effects after a period of training at 100% training load. Very intensive training shifted the CV autonomic modulation from PNS toward SNS predominance. Increases were reported in all components of HRV after a 1-year exercise training programme in children who initially had low HRV [60]. In 2001 Pigozzi et al., [61] found that a 5-week exercise training period in female athletes increased the sympathetic nervous system (SNS) cardiac modulation, which may coexist with relatively reduced or unaffected vagal modulation. Gulli et al., [62] reported increased LF reactivity (SNS) and BRS after a moderate aerobic training programme in older women, while Goldsmith et al., [63] noted that, although exercise training may increase PNS activity, studies report conflicting results.

Examples of Reports on Exercise and HRV Literature after 2005

A trend indicating increased resting vagal cardiac control is visible in reports on exercise induced changes measured by HRV [73, 74, 78, 79, 80, 81], with overall increased HRV [69, 71, 72, 75], accompanied by a possible decrease in ↓sympathetic activity [66, 67, 73]. Studies reporting no effect on HRV markers [65, 76, 77], are few and seems to be linked to the exercise intervention intensity and also the specific type of exercise intervention. For example Tai Chi conditioning and resistance training did not show significant changes in HRV indicator values [76].

In 2005 Sandercock et al., reviewed existing literature and came to the conclusion that significant exercise induced increases in RR interval and HF power are influenced by age and suggest that training bradycardia is caused by factors other than just increased vagal modulation [78]. Intervention results published in 2007 Sandercock et al., showed increases in sympathetic and parasympathetic HRV indicators after an eight week rehabilitation program [80]. A review by De Meerman and Stein (2006) reported the potential benefit of increasing or maintaining fitness in order to slow the decline of parasympathetic control of HR with normal aging [84]. Gademan et al., concluded that exercise has beneficial direct and reflex sympatho-inhibitory effects in chronic heart failure (2007) [85]. Montano et al., (2009) commented on moderate exercise training that may result in overall improvement in cardiac vagal control and reduced sympathetic activation in hypertensive patients who feature clear signs of elevated sympathetic activity [86]. According to Billman et al., endurance training alter autonomic nervous system activity by an apparent increase in cardiac parasympathetic tone coupled with decreases in sympathetic activity [83]. They suggested that the training bradycardia in both healthy subjects and patients with cardiovascular disease merits further investigation. A review by Routledge et al., (2010) on the use of exercise therapy as a method of HRV modification in clinical populations, reported that a shift toward greater vagal modulation may positively affect the prognosis of these individuals [73].

Many of the above mentioned reports (Table 1) and citations were based on supine HRV indicator values using only time domain and frequency domain analysis techniques.

Many factors in HRV analysis have the potential to lead to inconsistencies in results. Some studies used non-homogeneous participant groups with regard to age, gender and BMI, while, in a number of manuscripts, such information is not even mentioned. Factors generally not taken into consideration include baseline blood pressure, blood cholesterol, diet, fitness and other physiological characteristics. Other factors that could have an influence include the duration and intensity [37] of the training programs, as well as the type of exercise (endurance or resistance) [35]. When developing standardised procedures, inter-individual differences, duration and intensity of the exercise program, and the choice and implementation of a specific variability analysis technique should be carefully planned. Note should be taken of the specific techniques used when trying to compare values obtained by different laboratories. It may be incorrect to compare ANS results from publications where different techniques were employed. In addition to the type of analytical techniques used, elements in the practical implementation could very well also have an influence. Differences in tachogram length and period of recording used for analysis may contribute to controversies. The Task Force recommended that sampling time (tachogram) for short term HRV analysis should be 5 minutes [19], but different time windows are often selected by different authors, for example: 2 minutes, 5 minutes, 10 minutes, 15 minutes. HRV is known to be often non-normally (positively skewed) distributed. However non-parametric analytical techniques are sometimes used to analyse the data [66]. This may contribute to erroneous assumptions of statistical significance. Another possible explanation for conflicting results is that the individual's response may be greatly influenced by the baseline cardiovascular autonomic function, thus producing large inter-subject variation in the conventional non-spectral and spectral measures of cardiovascular variability.

Most studies incorporated in Table 1, used traditional measures of variability, such as time and frequency domain analysis. However, it is known that non-linear phenomena are also involved in cardiovascular control [65]. Therefore, it is of paramount importance that studies, using HRV as indicator of exercise induced changes in the ANS, should include analysis techniques that acknowledge this fact and non-linear measurements should be reported together with traditional measures. Examples of techniques that measure these aspects include the measurement of fractal scaling components (describes the fractal-like correlation properties of R-R interval data) and ApEn (quantifies the amount of complexity in the time series data) [65]. Another technique is the Poincaré plot where The RR intervals of the tachograms are plotted as a function of the preceding intervals. The Poincaré plot, a non-linear method of HRV quantification, is explained and used in Section 2 of this chapter.

The above overview demonstrates the wide variety of results published on the effect of training on the ANS as measured by cardiovascular variability indicators. It is clear from the results that standardization and refinement of these measuring tools are essential to produce repeatable results that can be used as references in other studies. This is necessary as these measurements are increasingly employed in studies ranging from investigations of central autonomic regulation; to studies exploring the link between psychological processes and physiological functioning; to the indication of ANS activity in response to exercise, training and overtraining. Much more research needs to be done to fully describe and accurately quantify the effect of exercise on the ANS.

In summary it can be said that the majority of recent review articles and individual research reports indicate increases in resting vagal cardiac control after exercise interventions as measured by HRV [73, 78, 79, 80, 81]. However, little is known about the influence of exercise on standing HRV or sympathetic cardiac control [79]. Claims of lower exercise induced sympathetic outflow as measured by HRV remains controversial as there is no single HRV indicator that represents pure sympathetic outflow [83].

The fact that the complex nature of the interaction between ANS function and exercise may not be fully explained by only one or two HRV indicators, neither by one position (such as the supine position), is not realized by many researchers in the field and may contribute to inconsistent results. In the supine position cardiac control is mainly controlled by vagal outflow, while during an orthostatic stressor the ANS balance is tipped towards sympathetic control [82]. As most reported exercise induced changes in RR intervals are measured only in the supine position, these changes may not depict the complete picture of exercise induced changes in the ANS. Measurements taken in the standing position may reveal important information on the sympathetic branch of the ANS that is not evident in the supine position.

References

[1] R.J. Shepard and G.J. Balady. Exercise as cardiovascular therapy. *Circulation.* 99, 963-972 (1999).

[2] M. Pagani, V.K. Somers and R. Furlan. Changes in autonomic regulation induced by physical training in mild hypertension. *Hypertension.*;12, 600-610 (1988).

[3] A.J.S. Coats, S. Adamopoulos an A. Radaelli. Controlled trial of physical training in chronic heart failure: exercise performance, hemodynamics, ventilation and autonomic function. *Circulation.* 85, 2119-213 (1992).

[4] G. Malfatto, M. Facchiniand L. Sala. Effects of cardiac rehabilitation and betha-blocker therapy on heart rate variability after first acute myocardial infarction. *Am. J. Cardiol.* 81, 834-840 (1998).

[5] US Department of Health and Human Services: Physical activity and health: a report of the Surgeon General. Atlanta, US Department of Health and Human Services, Centers for Disease Control and Prevention, National Center for Chronic Disease Prevention and Health Promotion. 1996.

[6] S.N. Blair, H.W Kohl, R.S. Paffenbarger, D.G. Clark, K. Cooper and L.W. Gibbons. Physical fitness and all-cause mortality. *JAMA.* 262(3), 2395–2401 (1989).

[7] Roy J. Shephard Exercise as Cardiovascular Therapy. Circulation. 1999;99:963-972.

[8] Mittelman MA, Maclure M, Tofler GH, Sherwood JB, Goldberg RJ, Muller JE. Triggering of acute myocardial infarction by heavy physical exertion. *N. Engl. J. Med.* 1993;329:1677-1683.

[9] S.N. Willich, M. Lewis and H. Lowell. Physical exertion as a trigger of myocardial infarction. *N. Engl. J. Med.* 329, 1684-1690 (1993).

[10] L. Mont, A. Sambola and J. Brugada. Lone atrial fibrillation in vigorously exercising middle aged men: case-control study. *BJM.* 316:1784-1785 (1988).

[11] H. Heidbüchel, J. Hoogsteen and R. Fagard. High prevalence of right ventricular involvement in endurance athletes with ventricular arrythmias. *Eur. Heart J.* 24, 1473-1480 (2003).

[12] M. Pichot, F. Roche and J.M. Gaspoz. Relation between heart rate variability and training load in middle-distance runners. *Med. Sci. Sports Exerc.* 32,1729-1736 (2000).

[13] L Mont and J. Brugada. Endurance athletes: exploring the limits and beyond. *Eur. Heart J.* 24, 1469-1470 (2003).

[14] S. Akselrod, D. Gordon, F.A Ubel, D.C. Shannon, A.C. Berger and R.J. Cohen. Power spectrum analysis of heart rate fluctuation: a quantitative probe of beat-beat cardiovascular control. *Science*. 213, 220-222(1981).

[15] S.H. Boutcher and P. Stein. Association between heart rate variability and training response in middle-aged men. *Eur. J. Appl. Physiol.* 70, 75-80 (1995).

[16] Michalsen and G.J. Dobos. Heart rate reduction through lifestyle modification. *Eur. Heart J.* 26(7), 1806-1807 (2005).

[17] D.M. Sacknoff, G.W. Gleim, N. Stachenfield and N.L. Coplan. Effect of athletic training on heart rate variability. *Am. Heart J.* 127, 1275-1278(1994).

[18] K. Shin, H. Minamitani, S. Onishi and M. Yamazakih-Lee. Autonomic differences between nonathletes: spectral analysis approach. *Med. Sci. Sports Exerc.* 29, 482-1490 (1997).

[19] Task Force of the European Society of Cardiology and the North American Society of Pacing and Electrophysiology. Heart rate variability: standards of measurement, physiology interpretation and clinical use. *Circulation.* 93,1043-1065 (2006).

[20] Y. Yamamoto, R.L. Hughson and J.C. Peterson. Autonomic control of heart rate during exercise studied by heart rate variability spectral analysis. *J. Appl. Physiol.* 71(3), 1136-1142 (1991).

[21] H. Schachinger, M. Weinhaber, A. Kiss, R. Ritz and W. Langewitz. Cardiovascular indices of peripheral and central sympathetic activation. *Psychosom Med.* 63, 788-796 (2001).

[22] R. Zhang, K. Iwasaki, J.H. Zuckerman, K. Behbehani, C.G. Crandall and B.D. Levine. Mechanism of blood pressure and R-R variability: insights from ganglion blockade in humans. *J. Physiol.* 543, 337-348 (2002).

[23] M. Al-ani, S.M. Munir, M. White, J. Towend and J.H Coote. Change in R-R variability before and after endurance training measured by power spectral analysis and by the effect of isometric muscle contraction. *Eur. J. Appl. Physiol.* 74, 397-403 (1996).

[24] G. Bertinieri, M. di Rienzo, A. Cavallazzi, A.U. Ferrari, A. Pedotti and G. Mancia. A new approach to analysis of the arterial baroreflex. *J. Hypertens Suppl.* 3(3), S79-S81 (1985).

[25] G.R. Sandercock, D.A. Brodie and G.R.H. Sandercock. The use of heart rate variability measures to assess autonomic control during exercise. *Scand. J. Med. Sci. Sports.* 16(5), 302-313 (2006).

[26] T. Banach, M. Grandys, K. Juszczak., W. Kolasinska-Kloch, J. Zoladz, J. Laskiewicz and P.J. Thor. Heart rate variability during incremental cycling exercise in healthy untrained young men. *Folia Medica Cracov.* 45(1-2), 3-12 (2004).

[27] J.V. Freeman, F.E. Dewey, D.M. Hadley, D. Myers and V. Froelicher. Autonomic nervous system interaction with the cardiovascular system during exercise. *Prog. Cardiovasc Dis.* 48(5), 342-362 (2006).

[28] B. Eryonucu, M. Bilge, N. Guler and I. Uygan. The effect of autonomic nervous system activity on exaggerated blood pressure response to exercise: evaluation by heart rate variability. *Acta Cardiologica.* 55(3), 181-185(2000).

[29] D. Lucini, V. Trabucchi, A. Malliani and M. Pagani. Analysis of initial autonomic adjustments to moderate exercise in humans. *J. Hypertens.* 13(12), 1660-1663 (1995).

[30] M. Saito and Y. Nakamura. Cardiac autonomic control and muscle sympathetic nerve activity during dynamic exercise. *Jpn J. Physiol.* 45(6), 961-977 (1995).

[31] M.V. Kamath, E.L. Fallen and R. McKelvie. Effects of steady state exercise on the power spectrum of heart rate variability. *Med. Sci. Sports Exerc.* 23(4):428-434 (1991).

[32] Y. Arai, J.P. Saul, P. Albrecht, L.H. Hartley, L.S. Lilly, R.J. Cohen and W.S. Colucci. Modulation of cardiac autonomic activity during and immediately after exercise. *Am. J. Phys.* 256, H132-141 (1989).

[33] Y. Yamamoto, R.L. Hughson, J.C. Peterson. Autonomic control of heart rate during exercise studied by heart rate variability spectral analysis. *J. Appl. Physiol.* 71(3), 1136-1142 (1991).

[34] R. Perini and A. Veicsteinas. Heart rate variability and autonomic activity at rest and during exercise in various physiological conditions. *Eur. J. Appl. Phys.* 90(3-4), 317-325 (2003).

[35] K.S. Heffernan, E.E. Kelly, S.R. Collier and B. Fernhall. Cardiac autonomic modulation during recovery from acute endurance versus resistance exercise. *Eur. J. Cardiovasc Prev. Rehabil.* 13(1), 80-86 (2006).

[36] P. Terziotti, F. Schena, G. Gulli and A. Cevese. Post-exercise recovery of autonomic cardiovascular control: a study by spectrum and cross-spectrum analysis in humans. *Eur. J. Appl. Phys.* 84(3), 187-194 (2001).

[37] N. Hayashi, Y. Nakamura and I. Muraoka. Cardiac autonomic regulation after moderate and exhaustive exercises. *Ann. Phys. Anthropol.* 1(3), 333-338 (1992).

[38] G. Raczak, G.D. Pinna, M.T. La Rovere, R. Maestri, L. Danil´owicz-Szymanowicz, W. Ratkowski, M. Figura-Chmielewska, M. Szwoch and K. Ambroch-Dorniak. Cardiovagal. response to acute mild exercise in young healthy subjects. *Circ. J.* 69(8), 976-980 (2005).

[39] K.S. Heffernan, S.R. Collier, E.E. Kelly, S.Y. Jae and B. Fernhall. Arterial stiffness and baroreflex sensitivity following bouts of aerobic and resistance exercise. *Int. J. Sports Med.* 28, 197-203 (2007).

[40] S.J. Brown and J.A. Brown. Resting and post-exercise cardiac autonomic control in trained master athletes. *J. Physiol. Sci.* 57(1), 23-29 (2007).

[41] D. Lucini, M. Cerchiello and M. Pagani. Selective reductions of cardiac autonomic responses to light bicycle exercise with aging in healthy humans. *Autneu.* 110(1), 55-63 (2004).

[42] Figueroa, T. Baynard, B. Fernhall, R. Carhart and J.A. Kanaley. Endurance training improves post-exercise cardiac autonomic modulation in obese women with and without type 2 diabetes. *Eur. J. Appl. Phys.* 100, 437-444 (2007).

[43] D.K. Spierer, R.E. DeMeersman, J. Kleinveld, E. McPherson, R.E. Fullilove, A. Alba and A.S. Zion. Exercise training improves cardiovascular and autonomic profiles in HIV. *Clin. Auton Res.* 17, 341-348 (2007).

[44] A.E. Aubert, L. Vanhees, F. Beckers, B.O. Eijnde, Verheyden. Low-dose exercise training does not influence cardiac autonomic control in healthy sedentary men aged 55-75 years. *J. Sports Sci.* 24(11), 1137-1147 (2006).

[45] F.S. Martinelli, M.P.T. Chacon-Mikahil, L.E.B. Martins, R. Lima-Filho, M.A. Paschoal and L. Gallo. Heart rate variability in athletes and non-athletes at rest and during head-up tilt. *Braz. J. Med. Biol. Res.* 38(4), 639-647(2005).

[46] R.K. Sharma, K.K. Deepak, R.L. Bijlani and P.S. Rao. Short-term physical training alters cardiovascular autonomic response amplitude and latencies. *Indian J. Physiol. Pharmacol.* 48(2), 165-173 (2004).

[47] M. Buchheit and C. Gindre. Cardiac parasympathetic regulation: respective associations with cardiorespiratory fitness and training load. *Am. J. Phys-Heart Circulatory Phys.* 291(1), 451-458(2006).

[48] G. Raczak, L. Danilowicz-Szymanowicz, M. Kobuszewska-Chwirot, W. Ratkowski, M. Figura-Chmielewska and M. Szwoch. Long-term exercise training improves autonomic nervous system profile in professional runners. *Kardiologia Polska.* 64(2), 35-140 (2006).

[49] K. Okazaki, K. IwasakI, A. Prasad, M.D. Palmar, E.R. Martini and A. Arbab-Zadeh, et al., Dose-response relationship of endurance training for autonomic circulatory control in healthy seniors. *J. Appl. Phys.* 99(3), 1041-1049 (2005).

[50] R.C. Melo, M.D. Santos, E. Silva, R.J. Quitero, M.A. Moreno, M.S. Reis and I.A.Verzola, et al., Effects of age and physical activity on the autonomic control of heart rate in healthy men. *Braz. J. Med. Biol. Res.* 38(9),1331-1338(2005).

[51] R.L. Goldsmith, D.M. Bloomfield and E.T. Rosenwinkel. Exercise and autonomic function. *Coron Artery Dis.* 11(2), 129-135 (2000).

[52] R.L Goldsmith, J.T. Bigger Jr, D.M. Bloomfield and R.C. Steinman. Physical fitness as a determinant of vagal modulation. *Med. Sci. Sports Exerc.* 29(6), 812-817 (1997).

[53] A.M. Kiviniemi, A.M. Hautala, T.H. Makikallio, H.V. Huikuri and M.P. Tulppo. Cardiac vagal outflow after aerobic training by analysis of high-frequency oscillation of the R-R interval. *Eur. J. Appl. Phys.* 96(6), 686-692 (2006).

[54] W.H. Cooke, B.V. Reynolds and M.G. Yandl. Effects of exercise training on cardiovagal and sympathetic response to Valsalva's maneuver. *Med. Sci. Sports Exer.* 34(6), 928-935 (2002).

[55] F. Costes, F. Roche, V. Pichot, J.M. Vergnon, M. Garet and J.C. Barthelemy. Influence of exercise training on cardiac baroreflex sensitivity in patients with COPD. *Eur. Respir. J.* 23(3), 396-401(2004).

[56] K.D. Monahan, F.A. DInenno and H. Tanaka. Regular exercise modulates age-associated declines in cardiovagal baroreflex sensitivity in healthy men. *J. Phys.* 529(1), 263-271 (2000).

[57] J.B. Carter, E.W. Banister and A.P. Blaber. Effect of endurance exercise on autonomic control of heart rate. *Sports Med.* 33(1), 33-46(2003).

[58] F. Iellamo, J.M. Legramante, F. Pigozzi, A. Spataro, G. Norbiato, D. Lucini and M. Pagani. Conversion from vagal to sympathetic predominance with strenuous training in high-performance world class athletes. *Circulation.* 105(23), 2719-2724 (2002).

[59] A.J. Bowman, R.H. Clayton, A. Murray, J.W. Reed, M.M.F. Subhan and G.A. Ford. Effects of aerobic exercise training and yoga on the baroreflex in healthy elderly persons. *Eur. J. Clin. Invest.* 27(5), 443-449 (1997).

[60] N. Nagai, T. Hamada, T. Kimura and T. Moritani. Moderate physical exercise increases cardiac autonomic nervous system activity in children with low heart rate variability. *Childs Nerv. Syst.* 20(4), 215-200 (2004).

[61] F. Pigozzi, A. Alabiso and A. Parisi. Effects of aerobic exercise training on 24hr profile of heart rate variability in female athletes. *J. Sports Med. Phys. Fitness.* 41(1), 101-107 (2001).

[62] G. Gulli, A. Cevese, P. Cappelletto, G. Gasparini and F. Schena. Moderate aerobic training improves autonomic cardiovascular control in older women. *Clin. Auton Res.* 13(3), 196-222 (2003).

[63] R.L. Goldsmith, J.T. Bigger Jr, R.C. Steinman and J.L Fleiss. Comparison of 24-hour parasympathetic activity in endurance-trained and untrained young men. *J. Am. Coll. Cardiol.* 20(3), 552-558 (1992).

[64] A.J. Hautala, T.H. Makikallio and A. Kiviniemi. Cardiovascular autonomic function correlates with the response to aerobic training in healthy sedentary subjects. *Am. J. Phys-Heart Circulatory Phys.* 285(4), 52-60 (2003).

[65] I.D. Laoutaris, A. Dritsas, M.D. Brown, A. Manginas, M.S. Kallistratos, A. Chaidaroglou, D. Degiannis, P.A. Alivizatos and D.V. Cokkinos. Effects of inspiratory muscle training on autonomic activity, endothelial vasodilator function, and N-terminal pro-brain natriuretic peptide levels in chronic heart failure. *J. Cardiopulm Rehabil. Prev.* 28, 99–106 (2008).

[66] G.E. Billman. Cardiac autonomic neural remodeling and susceptibility to sudden cardiac death: effect of endurance exercise training. *AJP-Heart.* 297, H1171-H1193 (2009).

[67] Borghi-Silva, R. Arena, V. Castello, R.P. Simo˜es, L.E.B. Martins, A.M. Catai and D. Costa. Aerobic exercise training improves autonomic nervous control in patients with COPD. *Respir Med.* 103, 1503-1510 (2009).

[68] L. Soares-Miranda, G. Sandercock, H. Valente, S. Vale, R. Santos and J. Mota. Vigorous physical activity and vagal modulation in young adults. *J. Cardiovasc. Risk.* 16, 70 (2009).

[69] B. Sridhar, N. Haleagrahara, R. Bhat, A.B. Kulur, S. Avabratha and P. Adhikary. Increase in heart rate variability with deep breathing in diabetic patients after 12-month exercise training. *Tohoku J. Exp. Med.* 220, 107-113 (2010).

[70] V.A. Cornelissen, B. Verheyden, A.E. Aubert and R.H. Fagard. Effects of aerobic training intensity on resting, exercise and post-exercise blood pressure, heart rate and heart-rate variability. *J. Hum. Hypertens.* 24, 175–182 (2010).

[71] E. Kouidi, V. Karagiannis, D. Grekas, A. Iakovides, G. Kaprinis, A. Tourkantonis and A. Deligiannis. Depression, heart rate variability, and

exercise training in dialysis patients. *Eur. J. Cardiovasc. Prev. Rehabil.* 17(2), 160-167. (2010).
[72] C. Knoepfli-Lenzin, C. Sennhauser, M. Toigo, U. Boutellier, J. Bangsbo, P. Krustrup, A. Junge and J. Dvorak. Effects of a 12-week intervention period with football and running for habitually active men with mild hypertension. *Scand. J. Med. Sci. Sports.* 20, 72–79 (2010).
[73] F.S. Routledge, T.S. Campbell, McFetridge-Durdle and S.L. Bacon. Improvements in heart rate variability with exercise therapy. *Can. J. Cardiol.* 26(6), 303-312 (2010).
[74] C.T. Albinet, G. Boucard, C.A. Bouquet and M. Audiffren. Increased heart rate variability and executive performance after aerobic training in the elderly. *Eur. J. Appl. Physiol.* 109, 617–624 (2010).
[75] H. Riesenberg and A.S. Lübbe. In-patient rehabilitation of lung cancer patients—a prospective study. *SCC.* 18, 877–882 (2010).
[76] S. Sato, S. Makita, R. Uchida, S. Ishihara and M. Masuda. Effect of Tai Chi training on baroflex sensitivity and heart rate vaiability in patients with coronary heart disease. *Int. Heart J.* 51, 238-241 (2010).
[77] J.D. Kingsley, V. McMillan and A. Figueroa. The effects of 12 weeks of resistance exercise training on disease severity and autonomic modulation at rest and after acute leg resistance exercise in women with fibromyalgia. *Arch. Phys. Med. rehabil.* 91(10), 1551-1557(2010).
[78] G.R.H. Sandercock, P.D. Bromley and D.A. Brodie. Effects of Exercise on Heart Rate Variability: Inferences from Meta-Analysis. *Med. Sci. Sports Exerc.* 37(3), 433–439 (2005).
[79] A.J. Hautala, A.M. Kiviniemi and M.P. Tulppo. Review Individual responses to aerobic exercise: The role of the autonomic nervous system. *Neurosci. Biobehav. Rev.* 33, 107 (2009).
[80] G.R.H. Sandercock, R. Grocott-Mason and D.A. Brodie. Changes in short-term measures of HRV after eight weeks of cardiac rehabilitation. *Clin. Auton Res.* 17, 39-45 (2007).
[81] S.T. Laing, T.J. Gluckman, K.M. Weinberg, M.K. Lahiri, J. Goldberger. Autonomic Effects of Exercise-Based Cardiac Rehabilitation. *J. Cardiopulm. Rehabil.* 31(2), 87–91(2011).
[82] N. Montano, A. Porta, C. Cogliati, G. Costantino, E. Tobaldini, K.R. Casali and F. Iellamo. Heart rate variability explored in the frequency domain: a tool to investigate the link between heart and behavior. *Neurosci. Biobehav. R.* 33(2), 71-80 (2009).

[83] G.E. Billman. Cardiac autonomic neural remodelling and susceptibility to sudden cardiac death: effect of endurance exercise training. *Am. J. Physiol. Heart Circ. Physiol.* 297, H1171-H1193 (2009).
[84] R.E. De Meersman, P.K. Stein. Vagal modulation and aging. Biological Psychology. 74, 165–173 (2007).
[85] M.G.J. Gademan, C.A. Swenne, H.F. Verwey, A. Van der Laarse, A.C. Maan, H. Van de Vooren, J . Van Pelt, et al., Effect of Exercise Training on Autonomic Derangement and Neurohumoral Activation in Chronic Heart Failure. *Journal of Cardiac Failure.* 13(4), 294-303 (2007).
[86] N. Montano, A. Porta, C. Cogliati, G. Costantino, E. Tobaldini, K.R. Casali and F Iellamo. Heart rate variability explored in the frequency domain: a tool to investigate the link between heart and behavior. *Neurosci. Biobehav. R.* 33(2),71-80 (2009).
[87] M. Esler, N. Straznicky, N. Eikelis, K. Masuo, G. Lambert and E. Lambert. Mechanisms of sympathetic activation in obesity-related hypertension. *Hypertension.* 48, 787–796 (2006).
[88] G. Mancia, G. Grassi, C. Giannattasio, G. Seravalle. Sympathetic activation in the pathogenesis of hypertension and progression of organ damage. *Hypertension.* 34, 724–728(1999).
[89] N. Montano, A. Porta, C. Cogliati, G. Costantino, E. Tobaldini, K.R. Casali and F Iellamo. Heart rate variability explored in the frequency domain: a tool to investigate the link between heart and behavior. *Neurosci. Biobehav. R.* 33(2),71-80 (2009).

In: Cardiovascular System　　　　　ISBN: 978-1-62948-308-5
Editors: M. Oberfield and Th. Speiser　© 2014 Nova Science Publishers, Inc.

Chapter 5

Endoplasmic Reticulum Stress in Cardiovascular Disease

Dukgyu Lee and Marek Michalak[*]
Department of Biochemistry, University of Alberta,
Edmonton, Alberta, Canada

Abstract

The endoplasmic reticulum (ER), an elaborate network of membrane, is the cellular organelle supporting diverse cellular functions: protein synthesis and folding, synthesis of phospholipids and steroids, and regulation of calcium homeostasis. Environmental stimuli such as oxidative stress and ischemic insult, or the accumulation of unfolded and/or misfolded protein cause ER stress; as a result, ER stress activates the unfolded protein response (UPR) to deal with a disruption of ER homeostasis. In the cardiovascular system, ER stress is linked to the pathologic states include ischemia, pressure overload, hypertension, atherosclerosis, hypertrophy, dilated cardiomyopathy, and heart failure. The UPR process is composed of a group of signal transduction pathways that improve the accumulation of unfolded protein by inhibiting protein translation, induction of ER chaperones, and accelerating the degradation of unfolded proteins. The UPR is an adaptive response to cope with ER stress but, if unresolved, it can lead to apoptotic cell death. Therefore, the

---

[*] Correspondence to:Dr. M. Michalak, Department of Biochemistry, University of Alberta, Edmonton, Alberta, Canada T6G 2H7, Tel: 780-492-2256, Fax: 780-492-0886.

development of therapeutic interventions that target molecules of the UPR signaling pathway and ameliorate ER stress will be convincing strategies to treat cardiovascular disease and other related disorders. In this chapter, we will discuss the recent progress in understanding the UPR pathway in cardiovascular disease and its related healing potential.

Introduction

Cardiovascular disease is one of the most costly health problems in the developed world, albeit the treatment of heart failure has advanced remarkably [1]. Thus, research for the development of novel therapeutic interventions in cardiovascular biology is of imperative importance. The endoplasmic reticulum (ER) is a multifunctional organelle responsible for diverse cellular functions as follows: the synthesis, folding, and posttranslational modification of proteins; the synthesis of lipids and steroids; the storage and release of Ca^{2+}; and the regulation of gene expression and energy metabolism [2, 3]. The ER has additional cellular functions in the heart, for example, the cellular reticular network of cardiac cells supports ER housekeeping functions and the regulation of excitation-contraction coupling [4]. Disruption of the ER functions results in ER stress, and sustained or severe ER stress causes the cell to undergo apoptotic cell death. To cope with ER stress, the ER triggers the unfolded protein response (UPR) in the cell. Thus, the ER is a critical intracellular organelle that allows cells to deal with a variety of stresses. Recently, adaptive pathways of UPR signaling have been implicated in the pathology of human diseases such as cardiovascular diseases, neurodegenerative diseases, diabetes mellitus, and obesity [5-7]. In this chapter, we will focus on the current progress in ER stress and the UPR signaling pathway, particularly in cardiovascular diseases, and its implication on the development of potential therapeutic compounds targeting components of the UPR pathway.

Endoplasmic Reticulum

The ER was first described nearly 7 decades ago as a "lace-like reticulum" [8], and has been extensively investigated in the field of biology. As an elaborate network of membrane, the ER is tightly connected with many cellular organelles include the nucleus [9], mitochondria [10], Golgi apparatus, plasma membrane, peroxisomes, and lysosomes, as well as precisely communicating with those organelles to maintain cellular functions. The ER is involved in protein synthesis, folding, post-translational modification [11]; and the synthesis of phospholipids and steroids on the cytosolic side of the ER membrane. To achieve proper folding of newly synthesized polypeptides in the secretory pathway, the ER contains several molecular chaperones including BiP/GRP78, calreticulin, and calnexin, and folding enzymes such as protein disulfide isomerase (PDI), ERp72, and ERp57. Furthermore, the ER is a major Ca^{2+} storage organelle and it regulates Ca^{2+} release into the cytosol by the inositol triphosphate (IP_3) receptor and Ca^{2+} channel, and consequently re-uptake of Ca^{2+} by the sarco/endoplasmic reticulum Ca^{2+} ATPase (SERCA). Both protein quality control and Ca^{2+}-regulated signal transduction by the ER require a high concentration of Ca^{2+} and tight regulation of Ca^{2+} in the lumen. In addition, an oxidizing environment in the ER lumen is critical for the formation of disulfide bonds that are required for the proper folding of proteins. As a consequence of these distinct environments, the ER is an important organelle that can detect and integrate incoming signals, generate outgoing signals in response to environmental changes, specifically perturb Ca^{2+} homeostasis or change the intraluminal redox states.

The Unfolded Protein Response Pathway

Numerous intrinsic and extrinsic factors: accumulation of unfolded/misfolded protein, oxidative stress, production of reactive oxygen species (ROS), Ca^{2+} and metabolite starvation, and viral infection, elicit ER stress. When ER stress occurs, three distinct ER transmembrane proteins are activated to trigger the UPR process (Fig. 1). These three sensor proteins are inositol-requiring enzyme 1 (IRE1), the ER kinase dsRNA-activated protein kinase-like ER kinase (PERK), and activating transcription factor 6 (ATF6). These proteins have their N-terminus inside the lumen of the ER and C-terminus in the cytosol except ATF6. In the unstressed (normal) state, these proteins interact with glucose-regulate protein 78-kDa (BiP/GRP78) when unfolded proteins accumulate in the ER lumen, BiP/GRP78 dissociates from these proteins to allow their dimerization and thereby initiation of the UPR (Fig. 1) [12].

IRE1 is a type I ER transmembrane protein consisting of a serine-threonine kinase module and an endoribonuclease domain in its cytoplasmic region. Activation of IRE1 by accumulation of unfolded protein, releases

BiP/GRP78 causes homodimerization and elicits endoribonuclease activity that specifically excises a 26-nucleotide intron from constitutively expressed X-box binding protein (XBP1) mRNA to generate spliced XBP1 (XBP1s). XBP1s binds to ER stress response elements I [ERSE-I: CCAAT(N9)CCACG] [13] and II [ERSE-II: ATTGG(N1)CCACG] [14], the UPR element (UPRE: TGACGTGG/A) [15], and cAMP-response element [CRE: TGACGT(C/A)(G/A) [16], to induce expression of diverse chaperone genes. Targeted disruption of the XBP1 gene results in embryonic lethality resulting from a developmental defect during cardiogenesis [17]. A dominant-negative form of XBP1 inhibits the XBP1-dependent arm of the UPR, leading to an increase in cardiomyocyte apoptosis during hypoxia [18]. Recently, it was found that the expression of brain natriuretic peptide (BNP) can be regulated by XBP1s through a novel AP1/CRE-like element in cardiomyocytes [19]. In addition, the regulatory subunits of phosphatidylinositol 3-kinase (PI$_3$K), p85α and p85β, interact with XBP1 and increase its translocation to nucleus. The interaction between PI$_3$K and XBP1s is absent in ob/ob mice, resulting in a defect in both the translocation of XBP1s and the regulation of ER stress [20]. These findings imply that XBP1s regulates gene expression in both the UPR and non-UPR states. Besides, IRE1α interacts with the tumor necrosis factor (TNF) receptor-associated factor (TRAF) 2, which leads to the activation of an apoptosis signal-regulating kinase (ASK) 1 [21, 22] and caspase 12 [23, 24]. This ASK1 pathway contributes to the development of heart and neurodegenerative diseases [25, 26]. These discoveries also demonstrate that IRE1α can mediate cell death signaling in the ER stress condition.

PERK is a serine threonine kinase that phosphorylates eukaryotic translation initiation factor (eIF) 2α on ER stress, which results in the inhibition of global translation, and reduces protein load in the ER lumen. But, there is one exception for translation inhibition by PERK. ATF4 is a transcription factor and binds to the promoter of GADD34, the regulatory subunit of the phosphatase that dephosphorylates eIF2α and restores cap-dependent translation [27]. Under normal condition, PERK activity is inhibited by prolyl hydroxylase, but when the activity of prolyl hydroxylase is constrained by hypoxic condition, post-ischemic infarct size of the heart is decreased by the activation of PERK activity [28]. CCAAT/enhancer-binding protein homologous protein (CHOP) is a proapoptotic transcription factor that is modulated by the ATF4 factor in the PERK pathway [7, 29].

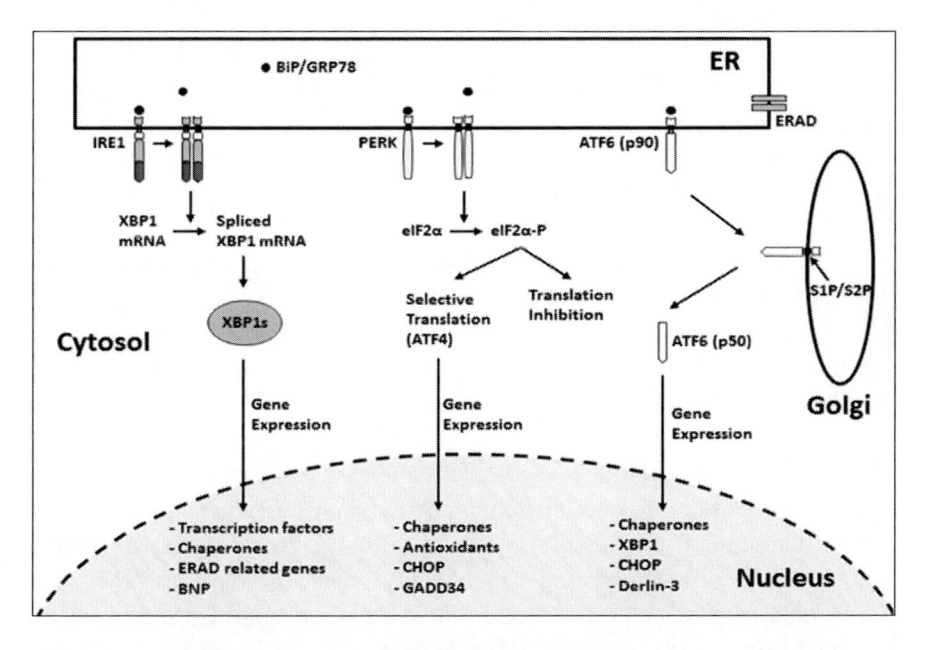

Figure 1. The UPR pathway. IRE1 and PERK are type I transmembrane proteins, and their N-terminal domains and C-terminal domains are located in the ER lumen and cytosol, respectively. IRE1 has both a Ser/Thr kinase domain for auto-phosphorylation and a RNase domain for endoribonuclease activity in cytoplasmic region. As well IRE1α is expressed ubiquitously, but the expression of IRE1β is restricted to the gut. PERK also has a Ser/Thr kinase domain to phosphorylate eIF2α and inhibit global protein translation. ATF6 is synthesized as a 90-kDa type II transmembrane protein with its N-terminal domain located in the cytosol. Upon ER stress, ATF6 is translocated to Golgi complex and cleaved by S1P and S2P proteases to produce an active 50-kDa ATF6. As an ER stress sensor, BiP/GRP78 maintains binding with these three transducers (IRE1, PERK, and ATF6) in the unstressed (normal) condition. Under ER stress, BiP/GRP78 dissociates from three ER transducers including IRE1, PERK, and ATF6, to allow their activation. A transmembrane IRE1 dimerizes, and leads to the activation of endoribonuclease activity that specifically cleaves the mRNA encoding the transcription factor XBP1. This unusual splicing event is required for translation of active XBP1s to bind to the ERSE or UPRE sequence of many UPR target genes including BiP/GRP78 and calreticulin. Activated (dimerized) PERK phosphorylates eIF2α, and this phosphorylated eIF2α switches off global protein translation, as well as induces the selective translation of a transcription factor, ATF4, to activate the expression of diverse UPR target genes including antioxidant genes. ATF6 (p90) translocates from the ER to the Golgi, in which ATF6 (p90) is cleaved by S1P and S2P proteases to yield a transcriptionally active ATF6 (p50). ATF6 (p50) activates a subset of UPR target genes include XBP1 and CHOP. Furthermore, unfolded/misfolded ER proteins are exported from the ER to cytosol by ERAD pathway, and degraded by the proteasome.

CHOP induces cell death through repression of antiapoptotic B-cell lymphoma-2 (Bcl-2) and BCL2/adenovirus E1B 19 kDa protein-interacting protein (Bnip3) expression in cardiomyocytes [30]. In addition, CHOP mediates the induction and translocation of Bim, a proapoptotic BH3-only protein of the Bcl-2 protein family, to the ER membrane in ER stress conditions [31].

ATF6 (p90) is an ER transmembrane transducer for ER stress. When BiP/GRP78 is released from ATF6, ATF6 is translocated from the ER to the Golgi and then cleaved by site-1 protease (S1P) and site-2 protease (S2P) to produce active ATF6 (p50), a basic leucine zipper transcription factor. By binding to the promoter of UPR target genes, ATF6 (p50) activates the expression of chaperones including BiP/GRP78, ER-associated protein degradation (ERAD) proteins, and XBP1. ATF6 activity was increased in the murine heart after myocardial infarction (MI), and treatment of mice with ATF6 inhibitor, 4-(2-aminoethyl) benzenesulfonyl fluoride, caused reduced cardiac function and increased the mortality rate at 14 days after MI [32]. ATF6 both performs a crucial role during the the UPR process and maintains cardiac function under physiological conditions.

As part of the ER stress response, ERAD is a process where misfolded proteins are exported from the ER to the cytosol and degraded by the 26S proteasome after poly-ubiquitination (Fig. 1) [33]. In the ER, loss of function of ERAD causes the accumulation of misfolded proteins and triggers the UPR [34], and many of the ERAD components are induced by the ATF6 branch in the UPR pathway. Derlin-3, a retrotranslocation channel, is one of example of a protein induced early by the UPR in the ischemic heart [35].

ER Stress and Cardiovascular Disease

A number of research advancements revealed that ER stress has been implicated in the pathophysiology of cardiovascular diseases such as congenital heart disease, cardiac hypertrophy and dilation, heart failure, ischemic heart disease, hypertension, and atherosclerosis. Collectively, ER stress and cardiovascular disease are confidentially interconnected, and the UPR pathway for dealing with ER stress may present a critical strategy for potential therapy of cardiovascular disease.

The fetal gene program and cardiogenesis. Reactivation of the fetal gene program in the adult damaged heart by ischemia, hypoxia, hypertrophy, or any other stimuli protects the stressed cardiac tissue through remodeling of the heart to increase cardiac efficiency. Long-term expression of the fetal gene program, however, results in deleterious cardiac hypertrophy [36]. Interestingly, one of the features of fetal gene program activation is up-regulation of early cardiac-specific transcription factors include MEF2C, NFAT, GATA, and Nkx2.5. These transcription factors contain ER stress-dependent elements (ERSE or UPRE) in their promoter region, suggesting these factors as potential targets for regulation by ER stress [37-40]. Besides, the fetal gene program exhibits up-regulation of ER chaperons, including BiP/GRP78, GRP94, and calreticulin, during the early developmental stage followed by a decay in expression during cardiogenesis [41]. This observation supports that premise that developing cardiac tissues have increased protein synthesis and secretion, and may undergo ER stress remediation by allowing tissue growth to avoid cell death. But conversely, adult cardiac tissues show a significant increase in the expression of ATF6, caspase 7 and caspase 12 [41]. Therefore, ER stress may play a critical role in reactivation of the fetal gene program and cardiogenesis.

Cardiac Ca^{2+} and heart failure. Oxidative stress, hypoxia, and disruption of Ca^{2+} homeostasis found in cardiac failure enhance ER stress. In human patients with cardiac failure, the expression of BiP/GRP78 and splicing of XBP1 (XBP1s) are increased, implying that UPR activation is related with the pathology of heart failure [42]. Indeed, the expression of ATF4 mRNA, CHOP, and ubiquitinated proteins is also upregulated in human patients [30, 43]. The mice after transverse aortic constriction (TAC) developed cardiac hypertrophy (1 week) and heart failure (4 weeks). Stimulated activation of the UPR in both hearts concomitantly activates the expression of CHOP [42]. Therefore, these findings suggest that UPR activation is persistent in the heart subjected to pressure overload.

Recently, our group has shown that calreticulin, an ER Ca^{2+} binding protein, induces heart failure via dilated cardiomyopathy in the adult mouse heart [44]. This cardiac dysfunction comes from the perturbation of Ca^{2+} homeostasis in the ER of cardiomyocytes, causing remodeling of sarcoplasmic reticulum (SR) Ca^{2+}-handling proteins and an abnormal conduction system. Moreover, the transgenic mice expressing a mutant KEDL (Lys-Asp-Glu-Leu) receptor, a retrieval receptor for ER chaperones, showed disrupted recycling of misfolded proteins between the ER and the Golgi complex and enhanced expression of CHOP [45]. The transgenic mice also exhibited dilated cardiomyopathy without obvious phenotypes in other tissue, suggesting that the heart is sensitive to ER stress. For these reasons, disruption of Ca^{2+}

homeostasis and accumulation of misfolded proteins in the heart are vulnerable to ER stress, causing cardiac failure.

Ischemic heart diseases. Under ischemic condition, oxygen and nutrients are depleted, causing protein aggregation in the ER, and this substantially triggers ER stress and the UPR [46, 47]. Specifically, during MI, BiP/GRP78 protein expression is increased near the infarct site, but conversely, no increase is observed far away from the damage [18]. Upon hypoxia, ER stress and the UPR are activated and protect the myocytes from ischemic damage. In the heart, ischemia activates the ER stress response by inducing the ATF6 pathway of the UPR, triggering the upregulation of BiP/GRP78 to target the damage produced by oxygen and nutrient starvation [48]. However, ATF6 activation and BiP/GRP78 promoter activity are attenuated by reperfusion. The other example is from the transgenic mice, a cardiac-specific expression of ATF6, in ischemic/reperfusion (I/R) injury [49]. ATF6 transgenic hearts show improved functional recovery from *ex vivo* ischemia reperfusion (I/R) stress, significantly reduced apoptosis, and also exhibit increased expression of BiP/GRP78 and GRP94. In addition, Glembotski's group demonstrated that ATF6 activation induces a number of genes include MANF (mesencephalic astorocyte-derived neurotrophic factor) in cultured cardiomyocytes [50]. Alternatively, the addition of recombinant MANF to culture media protects the cardiac myocytes from I/R-mediated cell death, however, knockdown of endogenous MANF by microRNA increases cell death on I/R stress. Moreover, the expression of Derlin-3, a component of the ERAD pathway, is stimulated by activated ATF6, and gain of function of Derlin-3 enhances ERAD signaling, and therefore protects cardiomyocytes from stimulated ischemia-derived cell death [35]. These findings demonstrate that ATF6 of the UPR pathway plays an important role in cardioprotection on I/R injury.

On the other hand, Terai et al. showed that hypoxia induces CHOP expression and the cleavage of caspase 12, but this effect is significantly suppressed by pretreatment with an activator of AMP-activated protein kinase (AMPK) [51]. Also, ER stress induces the expression of PUMA, a proapoptotic component of the Bcl-2 family, in neonatal cardiomyocytes, and the suppression of PUMA expression causes inhibition of myocyte apoptosis induced by a pharmacological ER stressor [52]. Similarly, the targeted deletion of PUMA attenuates cardiomyocyte cell death and improves cardiac function during I/R injury [53]. Thapsigagin, a pharmacological ER stressor, induces tribbles (TRB) 3 expression in HL-1 cultured cardiomyocytes, and MI results in cardiac ER stress caused by the induction of TRB3 [54]. Moreover, cardiac-restricted overexpression of TRB3 sensitizes mice to infarct expansion and cardiomyocyte apoptosis in the infarct border zone after MI. Interestingly, an agent that inhibits TRB3 expression may lead to reduced pathological cardiac remodeling in patients [54].

Hypertension and Atherosclerosis. Hypertension is a major risk factor for diverse cardiovascular diseases such as stroke, MI, or heart failure. During hypertension, the vasculature undergoes ER stress and ROS production, which triggers vascular remodeling involve the activation of the kinase Rac, the Rac subfamily of the family Rho family of GTPases, and results in cellular growth and hypertrophy [55]. The activation of Rac results in the phosphorylation of the c-Jun N-terminal kinase (JNK) pathway and of the downstream transcription factor (CHOP) [56]. In a rat model of hypertension, prostatic androgen repressed message-1 (PARM-1) is upregulated along with ER stress-induced BiP/GRP78, leading to cardiac hypertrophy and heart failure [57]. Specifically, silencing of PARM-1 results in increased cardiomyocyte apoptosis and decreased ATF6 expression, whereas increased expression of PARM-1 in response to ER stress is cardioprotective [57]. Therefore, PARM-1 regulates the expression of ATF6 in response to ER stress in hypertensive heart disease. ER stress specifically leads to ATF4-dependent activation of CHOP, which increases cellular ROS by transcriptionally up-regulating ER oxidase 1 alpha (ERO1α), which catalyzes the reoxidation of PDI family proteins in the ER [58]. In particular, reoxidation of PDI leads to an excess of ROS and to hyperoxidizing conditions in the ER, escalating the amount of aggregated proteins and stimulating apoptosis [59]. Sustained ER stress elicits the signaling pathway to eliminate affected cells, and this response is also observed in dilated and ischemic cardiomyopathies, and is characterized by cardiomyocyte loss, ventricular remodeling, and reduced systolic function [60].

Atherosclerosis is chronic vascular disease, and is caused by the formation of multiple plaques, and an accumulation of cholesterol and macrophages within the arteries [61]. Moreover, ER stress is apparently increased in endothelial cells subjected to atherosclerosis-prone shear stress [62]. Dong *et al.* found that reduction of AMPKα2 increases ER stress and atherosclerosis *in vivo*, and supresses SERCA activity in endothelial cells [63]. Thus, this result suggests that the physiological functions of AMPK as a suppressor of ER stress through maintaining SERCA activity and intracellular Ca^{2+} homeostasis. ER stress-induced apoptosis is a key cellular event in the conversion of benign to vulnerable atherosclerosis plaques. Remarkably, macrophage and smooth muscle cells in atherosclerotic plaques produces abundant secretory proteins, which can induce ER stress in these cells [61]. In addition, a cause of macrophage death is the accumulation of free cholesterol in the ER, which leads to activation of the UPR and CHOP-induced apoptosis [64, 65]. Another study showed that the association between ER stress and plaque rupture in human samples exhibited a strong correlation between ER stress markers such as CHOP and BiP/GRP78 and ruptured atherosclerotic plaques in human coronary artery lesions [66], indicating that ER stress is likely involved in the development of plaque rupture in human patients.

UPR Components as Therapeutic Applications

One of the fundamental strategies to develop therapeutic agents in treating cardiovascular is the activation of the adaptive pathway or deactivation of the proapoptotic pathway of the UPR components such as ATF6, IRE1, XBP1s, and eIF2α, and proteasome of the ERAD components. Current therapeutic agents used to target the UPR pathway are described in Table 1.

Table 1. Therapeutic agents targeting UPR components

Agent	Mechanism	Reference(s)
Metformin	Reduction of ER stress by AMPK activation	[67-69]
BiP inducer X	BiP/GRP78 induction	[70]
Tauroursodeoxycholic Acid (TUDCA)	Chemical chaperone	[71, 72]
Sodium phenylbutyrate (PBA)	Chemical chaperone	[73, 74]
Curcumin	GRP94 induction	[75]
Sunitinb	IRE1 activation	[76]
Salubrinal	Prevention of eIF2α dephosphorylation	[77]
EN460	ERO1 inhibitor; ROS reduction	[78]
SB203580	CHOP phosphorylation	[79]
Pioglitazone	Reduction of ER stress	[80]
Isoproterenol	Proteasome activation	[81]

Conclusion

Unbalanced ER homeostasis triggers an activation of the UPR pathway in various disorders including cardiovascular disease. Although our knowledge has extensively advanced to recognize non-homeostasis of the ER, many issues are still remained to be resolved. To address these issues, we need novel scientific approaches from diverse fields such as the use of microRNAs and the development of chemical chaperones to reduce ER stress, to answer the following questions, 1) What is the molecular mechanism involved in the decision to proceed to the adaptive or proapoptotic pathway of the UPR? 2) How do we develop new pharmaceuticals to activate or deactivate components of the UPR to improve disease state? 3) How can we deliver the agent to the targeted area? A deepened understanding of the essential mechanisms of the UPR in cardiovascular disease will provide us with new drug targets and therapeutic interventions.

Acknowledgments

This work was supported by a grant-in-aid from the Canadian Institute of Health Research.

Reviewed by Paul Eggleton, Institute of Biomedical and Clinical Sciences, Peninsula College of Medicine and Dentistry, University of Exeter, EX1 2LU, U.K., Tel 01392 722920, Fax 01392 722926, paul.eggleton@pms.ac.uk.

References

[1] Tang WH, Francis GS. The year in heart failure. *Journal of the American College of Cardiology*. 2010;55:688-96.

[2] Stutzmann GE, Mattson MP. Endoplasmic reticulum Ca(2+) handling in excitable cells in health and disease. *Pharmacological reviews*. 2011;63:700-27.

[3] Braakman I, Bulleid NJ. Protein folding and modification in the mammalian endoplasmic reticulum. *Annual review of biochemistry*. 2011;80:71-99.

[4] Michalak M, Opas M. Endoplasmic and sarcoplasmic reticulum in the heart. *Trends in cell biology.* 2009;19:253-9.
[5] Groenendyk J, Sreenivasaiah PK, Kim do H, Agellon LB, Michalak M. Biology of endoplasmic reticulum stress in the heart. *Circulation research.* 2010;107:1185-97.
[6] Minamino T, Kitakaze M. ER stress in cardiovascular disease. *Journal of molecular and cellular cardiology.* 2010;48:1105-10.
[7] Kim I, Xu W, Reed JC. Cell death and endoplasmic reticulum stress: disease relevance and therapeutic opportunities. *Nature reviews Drug discovery.* 2008;7:1013-30.
[8] Porter KR, Claude A, Fullam EF. A Study of Tissue Culture Cells by Electron Microscopy : Methods and Preliminary Observations. *The Journal of experimental medicine.* 1945;81:233-46.
[9] The unfolded protein response in nutrient sensing and differentiation. *Nature reviews Molecular cell biology.* 2002;3:411-21.
[10] Hayashi T, Rizzuto R, Hajnoczky G, Su TP. MAM: more than just a housekeeper. *Trends in cell biology.* 2009;19:81-8.
[11] Anelli T, Sitia R. Protein quality control in the early secretory pathway. *The EMBO journal.* 2008;27:315-27.
[12] Bertolotti A, Zhang Y, Hendershot LM, Harding HP, Ron D. Dynamic interaction of BiP and ER stress transducers in the unfolded-protein response. *Nature cell biology.* 2000;2:326-32.
[13] Yoshida H, Haze K, Yanagi H, Yura T, Mori K. Identification of the cis-acting endoplasmic reticulum stress response element responsible for transcriptional induction of mammalian glucose-regulated proteins. Involvement of basic leucine zipper transcription factors. *The Journal of biological chemistry.* 1998;273:33741-9.
[14] Kokame K, Kato H, Miyata T. Identification of ERSE-II, a new cis-acting element responsible for the ATF6-dependent mammalian unfolded protein response. *The Journal of biological chemistry.* 2001;276:9199-205.
[15] Yamamoto K, Yoshida H, Kokame K, Kaufman RJ, Mori K. Differential contributions of ATF6 and XBP1 to the activation of endoplasmic reticulum stress-responsive cis-acting elements ERSE, UPRE and ERSE-II. *Journal of biochemistry.* 2004;136:343-50.
[16] Wang Y, Shen J, Arenzana N, Tirasophon W, Kaufman RJ, Prywes R. Activation of ATF6 and an ATF6 DNA binding site by the endoplasmic reticulum stress response. *The Journal of biological chemistry.* 2000;275:27013-20.

[17] Reimold AM, Etkin A, Clauss I, Perkins A, Friend DS, Zhang J, et al. An essential role in liver development for transcription factor XBP-1. *Genes & development.* 2000;14:152-7.
[18] Thuerauf DJ, Marcinko M, Gude N, Rubio M, Sussman MA, Glembotski CC. Activation of the unfolded protein response in infarcted mouse heart and hypoxic cultured cardiac myocytes. *Circulation research.* 2006;99:275-82.
[19] Sawada T, Minamino T, Fu HY, Asai M, Okuda K, Isomura T, et al. X-box binding protein 1 regulates brain natriuretic peptide through a novel AP1/CRE-like element in cardiomyocytes. *Journal of molecular and cellular cardiology.* 2010;48:1280-9.
[20] Park SW, Zhou Y, Lee J, Lu A, Sun C, Chung J, et al. The regulatory subunits of PI3K, p85alpha and p85beta, interact with XBP-1 and increase its nuclear translocation. *Nature medicine.* 2010;16:429-37.
[21] Urano F, Wang X, Bertolotti A, Zhang Y, Chung P, Harding HP, et al. Coupling of stress in the ER to activation of JNK protein kinases by transmembrane protein kinase IRE1. *Science.* 2000;287:664-6.
[22] Nishitoh H, Matsuzawa A, Tobiume K, Saegusa K, Takeda K, Inoue K, et al. ASK1 is essential for endoplasmic reticulum stress-induced neuronal cell death triggered by expanded polyglutamine repeats. *Genes & development.* 2002;16:1345-55.
[23] Nakagawa T, Zhu H, Morishima N, Li E, Xu J, Yankner BA, et al. Caspase-12 mediates endoplasmic-reticulum-specific apoptosis and cytotoxicity by amyloid-beta. *Nature.* 2000;403:98-103.
[24] Saleh M, Mathison JC, Wolinski MK, Bensinger SJ, Fitzgerald P, Droin N, et al. Enhanced bacterial clearance and sepsis resistance in caspase-12-deficient mice. *Nature.* 2006;440:1064-8.
[25] Yamaguchi O, Higuchi Y, Hirotani S, Kashiwase K, Nakayama H, Hikoso S, et al. Targeted deletion of apoptosis signal-regulating kinase 1 attenuates left ventricular remodeling. *Proceedings of the National Academy of Sciences of the United States of America.* 2003;100:15883-8.
[26] Homma K, Katagiri K, Nishitoh H, Ichijo H. Targeting ASK1 in ER stress-related neurodegenerative diseases. *Expert opinion on therapeutic targets.* 2009;13:653-64.
[27] Ma Y, Hendershot LM. Delineation of a negative feedback regulatory loop that controls protein translation during endoplasmic reticulum stress. *The Journal of biological chemistry.* 2003;278:34864-73.

[28] Natarajan R, Salloum FN, Fisher BJ, Smithson L, Almenara J, Fowler AA, 3rd. Prolyl hydroxylase inhibition attenuates post-ischemic cardiac injury via induction of endoplasmic reticulum stress genes. *Vascular pharmacology.* 2009;51:110-8.

[29] Ron D, Walter P. Signal integration in the endoplasmic reticulum unfolded protein response. *Nature reviews Molecular cell biology.* 2007;8:519-29.

[30] Fu HY, Okada K, Liao Y, Tsukamoto O, Isomura T, Asai M, et al. Ablation of C/EBP homologous protein attenuates endoplasmic reticulum-mediated apoptosis and cardiac dysfunction induced by pressure overload. *Circulation.* 2010;122:361-9.

[31] Puthalakath H, O'Reilly LA, Gunn P, Lee L, Kelly PN, Huntington ND, et al. ER stress triggers apoptosis by activating BH3-only protein Bim. *Cell.* 2007;129:1337-49.

[32] Toko H, Takahashi H, Kayama Y, Okada S, Minamino T, Terasaki F, et al. ATF6 is important under both pathological and physiological states in the heart. *Journal of molecular and cellular cardiology.* 2010;49:113-20.

[33] Hebert DN, Bernasconi R, Molinari M. ERAD substrates: which way out? *Seminars in cell & developmental biology.* 2010;21:526-32.

[34] Su H, Wang X. The ubiquitin-proteasome system in cardiac proteinopathy: a quality control perspective. *Cardiovascular research.* 2010;85:253-62.

[35] Belmont PJ, Chen WJ, San Pedro MN, Thuerauf DJ, Gellings Lowe N, Gude N, et al. Roles for endoplasmic reticulum-associated degradation and the novel endoplasmic reticulum stress response gene Derlin-3 in the ischemic heart. *Circulation research.* 2010;106:307-16.

[36] Frey N, Olson EN. Cardiac hypertrophy: the good, the bad, and the ugly. *Annual review of physiology.* 2003;65:45-79.

[37] Potthoff MJ, Olson EN. MEF2: a central regulator of diverse developmental programs. *Development.* 2007;134:4131-40.

[38] Jamali M, Rogerson PJ, Wilton S, Skerjanc IS. Nkx2-5 activity is essential for cardiomyogenesis. *The Journal of biological chemistry.* 2001;276:42252-8.

[39] van Rooij E, Doevendans PA, de Theije CC, Babiker FA, Molkentin JD, de Windt LJ. Requirement of nuclear factor of activated T-cells in calcineurin-mediated cardiomyocyte hypertrophy. *The Journal of biological chemistry.* 2002;277:48617-26.

[40] Patient RK, McGhee JD. The GATA family (vertebrates and invertebrates). *Current opinion in genetics & development.* 2002;12:416-22.
[41] Papp S, Zhang X, Szabo E, Michalak M, Opas M. Expression of endoplasmic reticulum chaperones in cardiac development. *The open cardiovascular medicine journal.* 2008;2:31-5.
[42] Okada K, Minamino T, Tsukamoto Y, Liao Y, Tsukamoto O, Takashima S, et al. Prolonged endoplasmic reticulum stress in hypertrophic and failing heart after aortic constriction: possible contribution of endoplasmic reticulum stress to cardiac myocyte apoptosis. *Circulation.* 2004;110:705-12.
[43] Weekes J, Morrison K, Mullen A, Wait R, Barton P, Dunn MJ. Hyperubiquitination of proteins in dilated cardiomyopathy. *Proteomics.* 2003;3:208-16.
[44] Lee D, Oka T, Hunter B, Robinson A, Papp S, Nakamura K, et al. Calreticulin induces dilated cardiomyopathy. *PloS one.* 2013;8:e56387.
[45] Hamada H, Suzuki M, Yuasa S, Mimura N, Shinozuka N, Takada Y, et al. Dilated cardiomyopathy caused by aberrant endoplasmic reticulum quality control in mutant KDEL receptor transgenic mice. *Molecular and cellular biology.* 2004;24:8007-17.
[46] Glembotski CC. The role of the unfolded protein response in the heart. *Journal of molecular and cellular cardiology.* 2008;44:453-9.
[47] Szegezdi E, Duffy A, O'Mahoney ME, Logue SE, Mylotte LA, O'Brien T, et al. ER stress contributes to ischemia-induced cardiomyocyte apoptosis. *Biochemical and biophysical research communications.* 2006;349:1406-11.
[48] Doroudgar S, Thuerauf DJ, Marcinko MC, Belmont PJ, Glembotski CC. Ischemia activates the ATF6 branch of the endoplasmic reticulum stress response. *The Journal of biological chemistry.* 2009;284:29735-45.
[49] Martindale JJ, Fernandez R, Thuerauf D, Whittaker R, Gude N, Sussman MA, et al. Endoplasmic reticulum stress gene induction and protection from ischemia/reperfusion injury in the hearts of transgenic mice with a tamoxifen-regulated form of ATF6. *Circulation research.* 2006;98:1186-93.
[50] Tadimalla A, Belmont PJ, Thuerauf DJ, Glassy MS, Martindale JJ, Gude N, et al. Mesencephalic astrocyte-derived neurotrophic factor is an ischemia-inducible secreted endoplasmic reticulum stress response protein in the heart. *Circulation research.* 2008;103:1249-58.

[51] Terai K, Hiramoto Y, Masaki M, Sugiyama S, Kuroda T, Hori M, et al. AMP-activated protein kinase protects cardiomyocytes against hypoxic injury through attenuation of endoplasmic reticulum stress. *Molecular and cellular biology.* 2005;25:9554-75.

[52] Nickson P, Toth A, Erhardt P. PUMA is critical for neonatal cardiomyocyte apoptosis induced by endoplasmic reticulum stress. *Cardiovascular research.* 2007;73:48-56.

[53] Toth A, Jeffers JR, Nickson P, Min JY, Morgan JP, Zambetti GP, et al. Targeted deletion of Puma attenuates cardiomyocyte death and improves cardiac function during ischemia-reperfusion. *American journal of physiology Heart and circulatory physiology.* 2006;291:H52-60.

[54] Avery J, Etzion S, DeBosch BJ, Jin X, Lupu TS, Beitinjaneh B, et al. TRB3 function in cardiac endoplasmic reticulum stress. *Circulation research.* 2010;106:1516-23.

[55] Gregg D, Rauscher FM, Goldschmidt-Clermont PJ. Rac regulates cardiovascular superoxide through diverse molecular interactions: more than a binary GTP switch. *American journal of physiology Cell physiology.* 2003;285:C723-34.

[56] Brenner B, Koppenhoefer U, Weinstock C, Linderkamp O, Lang F, Gulbins E. Fas- or ceramide-induced apoptosis is mediated by a Rac1-regulated activation of Jun N-terminal kinase/p38 kinases and GADD153. *The Journal of biological chemistry.* 1997;272:22173-81.

[57] Isodono K, Takahashi T, Imoto H, Nakanishi N, Ogata T, Asada S, et al. PARM-1 is an endoplasmic reticulum molecule involved in endoplasmic reticulum stress-induced apoptosis in rat cardiac myocytes. *PloS one.* 2010;5:e9746.

[58] Gross E, Sevier CS, Heldman N, Vitu E, Bentzur M, Kaiser CA, et al. Generating disulfides enzymatically: reaction products and electron acceptors of the endoplasmic reticulum thiol oxidase Ero1p. *Proceedings of the National Academy of Sciences of the United States of America.* 2006;103:299-304.

[59] McCullough KD, Martindale JL, Klotz LO, Aw TY, Holbrook NJ. Gadd153 sensitizes cells to endoplasmic reticulum stress by down-regulating Bcl2 and perturbing the cellular redox state. *Molecular and cellular biology.* 2001;21:1249-59.

[60] Dorn GW, 2nd. Apoptotic and non-apoptotic programmed cardiomyocyte death in ventricular remodelling. *Cardiovascular research.* 2009;81:465-73.

[61] Hansson GK. Inflammation, atherosclerosis, and coronary artery disease. *The New England journal of medicine.* 2005;352:1685-95.

[62] Feaver RE, Hastings NE, Pryor A, Blackman BR. GRP78 upregulation by atheroprone shear stress via p38-, alpha2beta1-dependent mechanism in endothelial cells. *Arteriosclerosis, thrombosis, and vascular biology.* 2008;28:1534-41.

[63] Dong Y, Zhang M, Liang B, Xie Z, Zhao Z, Asfa S, et al. Reduction of AMP-activated protein kinase alpha2 increases endoplasmic reticulum stress and atherosclerosis in vivo. *Circulation.* 2010;121:792-803.

[64] Feng B, Yao PM, Li Y, Devlin CM, Zhang D, Harding HP, et al. The endoplasmic reticulum is the site of cholesterol-induced cytotoxicity in macrophages. *Nature cell biology.* 2003;5:781-92.

[65] Devries-Seimon T, Li Y, Yao PM, Stone E, Wang Y, Davis RJ, et al. Cholesterol-induced macrophage apoptosis requires ER stress pathways and engagement of the type A scavenger receptor. *The Journal of cell biology.* 2005;171:61-73.

[66] Myoishi M, Hao H, Minamino T, Watanabe K, Nishihira K, Hatakeyama K, et al. Increased endoplasmic reticulum stress in atherosclerotic plaques associated with acute coronary syndrome. *Circulation.* 2007;116:1226-33.

[67] Quentin T, Steinmetz M, Poppe A, Thoms S. Metformin differentially activates ER stress signaling pathways without inducing apoptosis. *Disease models & mechanisms.* 2012;5:259-69.

[68] Jung TW, Lee MW, Lee YJ, Kim SM. Metformin prevents endoplasmic reticulum stress-induced apoptosis through AMPK-PI3K-c-Jun NH2 pathway. *Biochemical and biophysical research communications.* 2012;417:147-52.

[69] Sasaki H, Asanuma H, Fujita M, Takahama H, Wakeno M, Ito S, et al. Metformin prevents progression of heart failure in dogs: role of AMP-activated protein kinase. *Circulation.* 2009;119:2568-77.

[70] Kudo T, Kanemoto S, Hara H, Morimoto N, Morihara T, Kimura R, et al. A molecular chaperone inducer protects neurons from ER stress. *Cell death and differentiation.* 2008;15:364-75.

[71] Ozcan U, Yilmaz E, Ozcan L, Furuhashi M, Vaillancourt E, Smith RO, et al. Chemical chaperones reduce ER stress and restore glucose homeostasis in a mouse model of type 2 diabetes. *Science.* 2006;313:1137-40.

[72] Erbay E, Babaev VR, Mayers JR, Makowski L, Charles KN, Snitow ME, et al. Reducing endoplasmic reticulum stress through a macrophage

lipid chaperone alleviates atherosclerosis. *Nature medicine.* 2009;15:1383-91.
[73] Cudkowicz ME, Andres PL, Macdonald SA, Bedlack RS, Choudry R, Brown RH, Jr., et al. Phase 2 study of sodium phenylbutyrate in ALS. *Amyotrophic lateral sclerosis : official publication of the World Federation of Neurology Research Group on Motor Neuron Diseases.* 2009;10:99-106.
[74] Lee B, Rhead W, Diaz GA, Scharschmidt BF, Mian A, Shchelochkov O, et al. Phase 2 comparison of a novel ammonia scavenging agent with sodium phenylbutyrate in patients with urea cycle disorders: safety, pharmacokinetics and ammonia control. *Molecular genetics and metabolism.* 2010;100:221-8.
[75] Pal R, Cristan EA, Schnittker K, Narayan M. Rescue of ER oxidoreductase function through polyphenolic phytochemical intervention: implications for subcellular traffic and neurodegenerative disorders. *Biochemical and biophysical research communications.* 2010;392:567-71.
[76] Korennykh AV, Egea PF, Korostelev AA, Finer-Moore J, Zhang C, Shokat KM, et al. The unfolded protein response signals through high-order assembly of Ire1. *Nature.* 2009;457:687-93.
[77] Boyce M, Py BF, Ryazanov AG, Minden JS, Long K, Ma D, et al. A pharmacoproteomic approach implicates eukaryotic elongation factor 2 kinase in ER stress-induced cell death. *Cell death and differentiation.* 2008;15:589-99.
[78] Blais JD, Chin KT, Zito E, Zhang Y, Heldman N, Harding HP, et al. A small molecule inhibitor of endoplasmic reticulum oxidation 1 (ERO1) with selectively reversible thiol reactivity. *The Journal of biological chemistry.* 2010;285:20993-1003.
[79] Cheng WP, Wang BW, Shyu KG. Regulation of GADD153 induced by mechanical stress in cardiomyocytes. *European journal of clinical investigation.* 2009;39:960-71.
[80] Yoshiuchi K, Kaneto H, Matsuoka TA, Kasami R, Kohno K, Iwawaki T, et al. Pioglitazone reduces ER stress in the liver: direct monitoring of in vivo ER stress using ER stress-activated indicator transgenic mice. *Endocrine journal.* 2009;56:1103-11.
[81] Asai M, Tsukamoto O, Minamino T, Asanuma H, Fujita M, Asano Y, et al. PKA rapidly enhances proteasome assembly and activity in in vivo canine hearts. *Journal of molecular and cellular cardiology.* 2009;46:452-62.

In: Cardiovascular System
Editors: M. Oberfield and Th. Speiser
ISBN: 978-1-62948-308-5
© 2014 Nova Science Publishers, Inc.

Chapter 6

Renal Sympathetic Denervation for Resistant Hypertension: Rationale and Results

Tushar Sharma, Rishi Talwar,[*]
Reza Khosravani Goshtaseb, and Anjay Rastogi
University of California, Los Angeles

Abstract

Hypertension is a significant global cause of morbidity and mortality, affecting no less than 1 billion people worldwide. In the United States, it affects more than 1 in 3 individuals, and almost 2 in 3 individuals above age 65. Despite the use of multiple medications, a huge number of patients don't reach their desired clinical target. Historically, over activation of sympathetic nervous system has been considered as playing a part in the pathogenesis of essential hypertension, and the relation has been made clearer by the use of techniques like microneurography and noradrenaline spill-over measurements. Kidneys have been found to be of an importance cause of this sympathetic overactivity. Based on this, a novel technique of renal sympathetic denervation has been developed to treat resistant hypertension. The results so far have been encouraging and it certainly deserves further research. This review article discusses the

---

[*] Corresponding author: University of California, Los Angeles.

burden of hypertension, the evidence of sympathetic overdrive playing a role in its etiology, the role of kidneys and the rationale behind renal denervation. It further sheds light on the results achieved, the problems faced and the weaknesses with each study done. In the end, it focuses on the prospects of his technique and realms for future research.

Introduction

Hypertension affects approximately 1 billion people around the world. [1] It is the most commonly diagnosed condition in the United States, especially among those aged 60 years or above. Existing prevalence of HTN exceeds 1 in 3 individuals, whereas two thirds of those above 65 years age have hypertension. [2, 3] In addition to these staggering figures, a large number of patients may not have been identified, because HTN is often asymptomatic. The importance of hypertension as an independent risk factor for coronary events, stroke, chronic heart failure, ESRD, as well as age-related dementia has been well documented. [4, 5] There exists a linear relationship between cardiovascular mortality risk and HTN, with the risk doubling for every 20 mm Hg and 10 mm Hg increase in systolic and diastolic blood pressure respectively, above 115/75 mm Hg. [3] HTN is responsible for 7 million deaths worldwide annually. [1] Given the prevalence and severity of the adverse outcomes, improvements in treatment of HTN are sure to result in widespread health benefits as well as decrease the financial burden on the society as a whole.

The percentage of patients with systemic hypertension that is under control has increased over the last twenty years. This may be due to the multitude of anti-hypertensives that are available and/or increased public awareness of HTN and its dangerous sequelae among both patients and primary care providers. Despite this notable progress, figures suggest that only 25-35% of patients can be acknowledged as having blood pressures that stay within the desired clinical goal range. [6–9] Inappropriate therapy, inadequate dosing or treatment inertia on the part of health care providers, as well as nonadherence and nonpersistence with the prescribed therapy on the part of the patient, partly due to intolerance, are all major contributors to lack of blood pressure goal achievement. [3, 7–13] In addition, there exists a subgroup of patients that is unable to achieve adequate blood pressure reduction, despite using multiple medications, necessary diet, and lifestyle modifications. Resistant hypertension is defined as blood pressure that remains above the desired goal despite concurrent use of 3 or more anti-hypertensives of different classes, one of which is a diuretic. The exact prevalence of resistant hypertension has yet to be established. However, clinical trials suggest that it is not rare, possibly involving up to 20-30% of study participants. [5, 9, 14–17] Given the burden that all these forms of hypertension present, it is clear that new, safe, and efficacious modalities of treatment are the need of the hour.

Sympathetic Nervous System and Hypertension

Pourfois du Petit is often credited as the first to consider a neural component of control of blood vessel caliber. He demonstrated in 1727 that conjunctival vessels would dilate after section of the cervical sympathetic nerve fibers. [18] In 1840, Stelling concluded that the vasomotor nerves were sympathetic nerves from the central nervous system to the blood vessels. Bernard, Waller and Brown-Sequard showed these as the "pressor nerves" by demonstrating vasoconstriction with electrical stimulation of the cut nerves, accompanied by blood pressure elevation, and vasodilation on nerve section. [18] Von Euler, in 1946 demonstrated that the sympathetic transmitter was noradrenaline.

The "neurogenic hypothesis of hypertension" describes an imbalance in sympathetic and parasympathetic nervous systems as part of the pathophysiological development of essential hypertension. The hypothesis that abnormalities in the autonomic modulation of blood pressure homeostasis, i.e., sympathetic activation and parasympathetic inactivation, may be a part of the etiology of essential hypertension, has been tested repeatedly with favorable results. Considered the best rat model for human essential hypertension, the spontaneously hypertensive rat (SHR) has displayed evidence of an overactive sympathetic system. Both the level of turnover of noradrenaline in the pressor areas of the SHR's central nervous system and the vasoconstriction response to varied stimuli were found to be amplified. [19] Importantly, similar physiological alterations have been shown to occur in humans with essential hypertension. Encouraging results were further provided by this animal model when it was demonstrated that by denervating the kidneys or with chemical sympathectomy, the development of hypertension could be delayed or prevented. [20]

Measurement of plasma noradrenaline as a humoral marker of sympathetic activity was the dominant methodology through the 1970s, and an analytic review has shown that in about 40% of the studies employing plasma noradrenaline as a marker for sympathetic drive in patients with essential hypertension, high blood pressure was indeed associated with elevated plasma noradrenaline values. [21] In another analysis, it has been shown that the plasma levels of noradrenaline are 25-30% higher in patients with essential hypertension when compared to control patients. [22–25]

More recently, microneurographic recording of postganglionic sympathetic neural outflow to the skeletal muscle has provided evidence of marked sympathetic activation in hypertensive patients. [25–33] These studies have shown that firstly, the adrenergic overdrive is directly proportional to the severity of hypertension. This evidence suggests the possibility of a cause-and-result relationship. Secondly, sympathetic overactivity is a constant factor in various presentations of hypertension, including a) Borderline, mild to moderate and severe hypertension b) HTN affecting young, middle aged and elderly people c) Systodiastolic and isolated systolic HTN d) pregnancy induced HTN e) white coat and masked HTN and f) dipping, extreme dipping, non-dipping, and reverse dipping conditions. Thirdly, sympathetic activation is a peculiar feature of essential HTN, and is not as well appreciated in secondary hypertensive states. Finally, the studies point out that the magnitude of sympathetic overdrive seems to be augmented when the hypertensive state is complicated by presence of end organ damage like left ventricular hypertrophy or ESRD.

Critically, these studies also show that in many renal and cardiometabolic diseases, including hypertension, the level of sympathetic activity in the skin remains relatively normal while sympathetic outflow to muscle is simultaneously elevated. This suggests that the adrenergic overdrive in hypertension isn't homogenous throughout the body. The novel noradrenaline radiolabelling technique has enabled us to understand the regional patterns of sympathetic overdrive in hypertension better. In hypertension, there is potentiation of central, cardiac, and renal noradrenaline spillover. [34–39] Interestingly, renal noradrenaline spillover, on an average was found to be elevated two-to threefold, pointing towards the major role played by renal sympathetic nerves in the development of hypertension.

Role of Kidneys and Rationale for Renal Denervation

The sympathetic supply to the kidneys is through the renal sympathetic plexus, whose fibers course along the renal arteries to reach each kidney. These sympathetic nerves enter the kidneys in the walls of renal arteries, and affect the renal function in 3 ways: a) increase renin secretion through β_1 receptors, leading to activation of renin-angiotensin system b) enhance sodium and water reabsorption through α_{2B} receptors, and c) induce renal vasoconstriction with renal blood flow and glomerular flow rate reduction through α_{1A} receptors.

All these mechanisms lead to fluid retention and elevation of blood pressure. Renal sympathetic nerve stimulation causes elevated blood pressure in the canine model. [40] This observation seems to be further vindicated in a model of unilateral renal denervation in dogs treated by rapid injection of 6-hydroxydopamine into the renal artery with simultaneous collection of venous effluents to avoid systemic effects. [41] On the other hand, Angiotensin II acts on different levels, i.e., the kidney, the central nervous system as well as peripheral sites to induce noradrenaline release from sympathetic nerve terminals. [42, 43] The sympathetic system and RAAS thus appear to act via reciprocal potentiation. Long-term low dose angiotensin II infusion in rats produces a gradual increase in blood pressure, and kidney denervation in the same model partially prevented hypertension. [44] This illustrates the importance of both sympathetic overactivity and RAAS in the pathophysiology of hypertension. Kidney ischemia appears to be the most significant stimulus for central sympathetic activity and RAAS. [45] Even minimal kidney damage that may not affect kidney function can cause ischemic foci in the kidney, leading to activation of RAAS and the central sympathetic drive in parallel. Studies in rats have shown that even a minute lesion by injection of phenol into one kidney caused increased central sympathetic activity and hypertension. [46] Even in humans, sympathetic nerve activity in muscles is increased in CKD patients, but it is normal in bilaterally nephrectomized patients. [47, 48] The evidence suggests strongly that kidney disease is a clear trigger for sympathetic overactivity. Kidneys also control the RAAS and it has been shown that bilaterally nephrectomized patients have undetectable variability of the circulating RAAS components. [49] That the two work in congruence can also be inferred from the observation that the activity of both systems shifts in parallel with changes in fluid status. [50] Intravenous injection of angiotensin II has been shown to stimulate sympathetic nerve activity in muscles of humans. [51] Hence, a cause-and-effect relation seems to be present, although further research needs to be done to validate this hypothesis.

Keeping in mind that the overactive efferent renal sympathetic fibers lead to fluid retention and activation of RAAS, and that afferent renal fibers directly appear to cause central sympathetic overdrive in presence of even minimal kidney lesions, it makes logical sense to explore the use of renal sympathetic denervation to control hypertension. Various preclinical and human studies have accordingly been done, and the results have been encouraging.

Renal Denervation

Apart from the studies done in rats mentioned above, the safety and feasibility of transluminal sympathetic ablation have been investigated in larger animal models as well. Renal denervation successfully decreased blood pressure in swine with established hypertension being treated with deoxycorticosterone acetate. [10] The technique also attenuates systemic hypertension and sodium retention associated with obesity in dogs. [52] Of note, this procedure, via ablation of sympathetic nerves through a radiofrequency based catheter system in a swine model was not associated with clinically significant adverse renal findings 6 months after the procedure. [53] At the molecular level, a new study showed that renal denervation significantly reduced collagen content and the mRNA expression of collagen I and III, in addition to altering the expression of fetal gene programming in rats undergoing experimental aortic regurgitation, with the final effect of preventing albuminuria and glomerular podocyte injury when added to an angiotensin II type I receptor blocker, thus providing new insights into management of cardio-renal syndrome. [54] These preclinical studies, taken together emphasize the therapeutic potential of renal denervation, and point out the safety of the procedure.

Due to the appeal of the procedure, unselective sympatholytic surgery has also been practiced in humans since 1930s to treat severe hypertension, when oral pharmacological therapies were not available. The surgical approaches were mainly thoracic, abdominal or pelvic in order to achieve radical sympathetic denervation. [55] However, these methods were associated with high perioperative morbidity, mortality, and long-term complications, including severe orthostatic hypotension, orthostatic tachycardia, palpitations, breathlessness, anhidrosis, cold hands, as well as bladder dysfunction, intestinal disturbances, loss of ejaculation, sexual dysfunction, thoracic duct injuries, and atelectasis. Also, blood pressure reduction was inconsistent and observed in about only 50% of the cases. [56, 57] Hence, the procedure was largely abandoned with the arrival of effective and better tolerated anti-hypertensive drugs in the late 1950s and 1960s.

Recently the concept of renal denervation has seen a new interest after the development of far less side effect-prone method of catheter based endovascular radiofrequency ablation of renal sympathetic nerves. The technique resembles an ordinary arteriogram. Energy is generated by a radiofrequency generator and applied on various spots of the wall of renal arteries where both afferent and efferent renal nerves are located, thus destroying them.

Interestingly, physiological mechanisms for regulating electrolytes, volume status and adrenaline mediated stress responses are preserved. [58,59] This is consistent with the historical knowledge that a transplanted denervated human kidney maintains electrolyte and volume homeostasis. Of note, early clinical evaluation with this technique has mechanistically correlated sympathetic efferent denervation with decreased renal norepinephrine spillover, halving of renin activity and increased renal plasma flow, and suggests reduced central sympathetic drive through demonstration of reduced total body norepinephrine spillover and muscle sympathetic nerve activity. This establishes that the technique indeed ablates renal sympathetic nerves, and taken together with the reduction of blood pressure that has been seen, it reinforces the role of sympathetic overdrive in the pathophysiology of HTN.

Krum et al. were the ones to report the first proof-of-principle, non-randomized trial of therapeutic renal denervation in patients with resistant HTN. The trial included a cohort of 45 patients with resistant HTN (SBP ≥160 mmHg on ≥3 anti-HTN drugs, including a diuretic; eGFR ≥ 45 mL/min). After only 1 month of renal denervation, SBP and DBP had decreased by 14 mm Hg and 10 mm Hg respectively. By 12 month follow up, the decreases were 27 mm Hg and 17 mm Hg. The study provided the first evidence that ablation-induced renal denervation is safe and efficacious. [60]

Although limited by a lack of control group, suboptimal candidate exclusion criteria and small patient number, the study proved that further research was warranted, and inevitably led to the Symplicity HTN-1 trial that was indeed built upon the previous cohort by increasing the patient number. It was a series of pilot studies involving 153 patients aged 57±11 years. 31% had Diabetes type II. Baseline data included mean office blood pressure of 176/98±17/15 mmHg, mean of 5.1±1.4 anti-HTN medications, and an eGFR of 83±20ml/min/1.73m^2. The median procedure time was 38 minutes. Minor complications were reported in 4 cases, including 3 groin pseudoaneurysms and 1 renal artery dissection, all managed without further sequelae. Reductions of 22/10 mmHg, 27/14 mmHg, 29/14 mmHg and 31/16 mmHg have been reported at 6 months, 1 year, 2 years and 3 years, respectively. [61]

Furthermore, according to the data presented at the American college of Cardiology annual meeting 2012, the percentage of responders (defined as office SBP reduction≥10 mmHg) was 69%, 71%, 79%, 90% and 100% at 1 month, 6 months, 1 year, 2 years and 3 years. Also of note, among non-responders at 1 month, the response rate was 57% at 6 months, 64% at 1 year, 82% at 2 years and 100% at 3 years. Renal imaging at 6 months did not show any abnormalities and there were no significant adverse effects after 3 years of follow up. The data from Symplicity HTN-1 trial suggests that the magnitude of clinical response is significant and sustained through 3 years post-procedure, that the response may actually get potentiated with time in non-responders, and that the treatment effect was consistent across subgroups (age, diabetes status, and baseline renal function). The weaknesses in the trial are that it lacked a proper control group, had a small number of patients, the group of patients recruited was not clearly defined, and predictors of blood pressure response had not been identified.

The limitations have been addressed in the Symplicity HTN-2, a prospective, randomized controlled clinical trial that recruited similar cohort of patients to the HTN-1 trial. Of the 106 patients randomized, 52 were assigned for renal denervation and 54 acted as controls. In the end, 49 underwent RDN and 51 continued as controls. All kept on receiving their anti-HTN medications. In patients undergoing RDN, 1 renal artery dissection and 1 hospitalization due to hypotension were reported, both treated without further consequences. Besides, 1 femoral artery pseudoaneurysm, 1 post-procedural drop in BP, 1 urinary tract infection, 1 prolonged hospitalization for evaluation of paraesthesias, and 1 back pain were reported in the full cohort, all treated without sequelae At 6 months, patients randomized into the control group receiving antihypertensive medications alone had blood pressures that did not vary from baseline (+1/0 mmHg), while the RDN therapy plus antihypertensives treatment arm demonstrated a reduction in mean blood pressure (-32/-12 mmHg). [62]

The data for the latest 24 month follow up of all patients was presented at the American Cardiology Congress in March 2013. The original RDN treatment arm, the control crossover arm (the control group that underwent RDN after 6 months), and the combined cohort all achieved sustained blood pressure reductions of -29/-10 mmHg, -35/-13 mmHg, and -31/-11 mmHg respectively. [63] Similar to HTN-1, no vascular abnormalities were seen on renal imaging at 6 months. In both HTN-1 and HTN-2, there have been no serious device or procedure-related events, and the renal function has been maintained. Encouraged by the results shown by these two trials, a third in the series, the Symplicity HTN-3 trial has been designed. It is a prospective, randomized, masked procedure, single-blind trial. It aims to randomize 530 patients to RDN and control groups in a 2:1 ratio. Both the study patients and the research staff who assess the blood pressure will be blinded. [64] Another improvement over HTN-2 is that change in average 24-hour ambulatory blood pressure is a major secondary effectiveness end point, thus giving us a better idea about the daily variations in blood pressure before and after the procedure. Based on the successful results of its predecessors, this trial is also expected to bring in encouraging results.

Discussion

The studies indicate that there may be a single non-pharmacological strategy to address resistant hypertension, which we have not been able to address adequately. It also eliminates the requirement for the patients to be on polypharmacy throughout their lives, thus taking care of the problem of non-compliance. Although the procedure is costly today, it may prove to be cost-effective once the burden of life-long polypharmacy is taken into account. A cost-effectiveness analysis is mandated in this regard. Another benefit of this elegant procedure is that it gives us an insight into the pathophysiology of HTN. The fact that a single localized intervention has such profound systemic effects gives us another perspective into the role of kidneys and the sympathetic nervous system in the pathogenesis of various diseases.

In the future, research should concentrate on the safety and efficacy of this technique in other diseases like heart failure, CKD, sleep apnea, metabolic syndrome and obesity, since sympathetic overactivity seems to be important in these conditions as well. Whether the technique is safe and feasible in less severe HTN is another topic for research. It also presents with an opportunity to study the relation between insulin resistance and sympathetic overactivity, since studies seem to suggest the relation may be bidirectional. It will be interesting to find out exactly which subsets of patients are benefitted by the procedure. Since the technique may cause direct injury to the vascular endothelium and smooth muscle cells, whether and to what extent they play a role in the effects seen remains to be studied. Additional studies should attempt to quantify the role of afferent and efferent renal fibers in the blood pressure reduction, possibly by clarifying the extent to which changes in circulating volume and sodium and fluid homeostasis determine the hemodynamic mechanisms leading to the reduction. Efferent nerves may anatomically regrow leading to cancelling out of the effect to some degree, but afferent nerves are unlikely to. As the reduction in blood pressure has been sustained for more than 3 years, it possibly highlights the major role played by the afferents in the pathogenesis. Nevertheless, an eye should be kept out to look for any functional reinnervation of the efferents, and to what extent it alters the results, if at all. Blinded, randomized studies to monitor the response of sympathetic activity after RDN, possibly by studying the norepinephrine spillover or by microneurographic studies, are also warranted. Long term follow-up of the anatomy and morphology of renal arteries and kidneys after RDN are necessary, even though the current data makes the modality look safe. Any long term effects on kidney function should also be a subject for future studies. Finally, the ill effects of exposure to radiation during the procedure should be taken into account. The important thing to consider here is that a high percentage of patients with resistant hypertension are obese, and these are the people who require higher doses of radiation.

Conclusion

Through rigorous study and relentless research the complex relationship between the sympathetic nervous system and its modulation on blood pressure through the kidneys has gradually been revealed. From this knowledge, several pharmaceutical agents have been developed for the battle against hypertension: α-methyldopa, β-blockers, α-blockers, ACE inhibitors, moxonidine, and ARBs. Two commonly applied non-pharmacological therapies for HTN, aerobic exercise training and calorie restriction, inhibit the sympathetic nervous system and that is probably why these two seem to be the most effective among all non-pharmacological therapies. None of these however have turned out to be as effective as RDN. It has proven to be a safe, efficacious and feasible modality according to the data available till now, and may also prove to be cost-effective in the long run. Nevertheless, further larger studies for long term safety and efficacy of the procedure, its applications in other diseases and for providing clear indicators and precise parameters of successful renal artery ablation are most welcome and required.

References

[1] Go, AS; Mozaffarian, D;, Roger, VL; et al. Heart disease and stroke statistics--2013 update, a report from the American Heart Association. *Circulation*, 2013, 127(1), e6–e245. doi, 10.1161/ CIR.0b013e31 828124 ad.

[2] Kearney, PM; Whelton, M; Reynolds, K; Muntner, P; Whelton, PK, He, J. Global burden of hypertension, analysis of worldwide data. *Lancet*, 365(9455), 217–23. doi, 10.1016/S0140-6736(05)17741-1.

[3] Lewington, S; Clarke, R; Qizilbash, N; Peto, R; Collins, R. Age-specific relevance of usual blood pressure to vascular mortality, a meta-analysis of individual data for one million adults in 61 prospective studies. *Lancet*, 2002, 360(9349), 1903–13. Available at, http, //www.ncbi.nlm.nih.gov/pubmed/12493255. Accessed May 21, 2013.

[4] Whitworth, JA. 2003 World Health Organization (WHO)/International Society of Hypertension (ISH) statement on management of hypertension. *Journal of hypertension*, 2003, 21(11), 1983–92. doi, 10.1097/01.hjh.0000084751.37215.d2.

[5] Roger, VL; Go, AS; Lloyd-Jones, DM; et al. Heart disease and stroke statistics--2012 update, a report from the American Heart Association. *Circulation*, 2012, 125(1), e2–e220. doi, 10.1161/ CIR.0b013e318 23ac046.

[6] Lloyd-Jones, DM; Evans, JC; Levy, D. Hypertension in adults across the age spectrum, current outcomes and control in the community. *JAMA, the journal of the American Medical Association*, 2005, 294(4), 466–72. doi, 10.1001/jama.294.4.466.

[7] Ostchega, Y; Yoon, SS; Hughes, J; Louis, T. Hypertension awareness, treatment, and control--continued disparities in adults, United States, 2005-2006. *NCHS data brief*, 2008, (3), 1–8. Available at, http, //www.ncbi.nlm.nih.gov/pubmed/19389317. Accessed June 15, 2013.

[8] Egan, BM; Zhao, Y; Axon, RN. US trends in prevalence, awareness, treatment, and control of hypertension, 1988-2008. *JAMA, the journal of the American Medical Association*, 2010, 303(20), 2043–50. doi, 10.1001/jama.2010.650.

[9] Sarafidis, PA; Bakris, GL. Resistant hypertension, an overview of evaluation and treatment. *Journal of the American College of Cardiology*, 2008, 52(22), 1749–57. doi, 10.1016/j.jacc.2008.08.036.

[10] O'Hagan, KP; Thomas, GD; Zambraski, EJ. Renal denervation decreases blood pressure in DOCA-treated miniature swine with

established hypertension. *American journal of hypertension*, 1990, 3(1), 62–4. Available at, http, //www.ncbi.nlm.nih.gov/pubmed/2302330. Accessed June 15, 2013.

[11] Conlin, PR; Gerth, WC; Fox, J; Roehm, JB; Boccuzzi, SJ. Four-Year persistence patterns among patients initiating therapy with the angiotensin II receptor antagonist losartan versus other artihypertensive drug classes. *Clinical therapeutics*, 2001, 23(12), 1999–2010. Available at, http, //www.ncbi.nlm.nih.gov/pubmed/11813934. Accessed June 15, 2013.

[12] Rosendorff, C; Black, HR; Cannon, CP; et al. Treatment of hypertension in the prevention and management of ischemic heart disease, a scientific statement from the American Heart Association Council for High Blood Pressure Research and the Councils on Clinical Cardiology and Epidemiology and Preventi. *Circulation*, 2007, 115(21), 2761–88. doi, 10.1161/CIRCULATIONAHA.107.183885.

[13] Mancia, G; De Backer, G; Dominiczak, A; et al. 2007 Guidelines for the management of arterial hypertension, The Task Force for the Management of Arterial Hypertension of the European Society of Hypertension (ESH) and of the European Society of Cardiology (ESC). *European heart journal*, 2007, 28(12), 1462–536. doi, 10.1093/eurheartj/ehm236.

[14] Bibbins-Domingo, K; Chertow, GM; Coxson, PG; et al. Projected effect of dietary salt reductions on future cardiovascular disease. *The New England journal of medicine*, 2010, 362(7), 590–9. doi, 10.1056/NEJMoa0907355.

[15] Noda, K; Zhang, B; Iwata, A; et al. Lifestyle changes through the use of delivered meals and dietary counseling in a single-blind study. The STYLIST study. *Circulation journal, official journal of the Japanese Circulation Society*, 2012, 76(6), 1335–44. Available at, http, //www.ncbi.nlm.nih.gov/pubmed/22739083. Accessed June 15, 2013.

[16] Persell, SD. Prevalence of resistant hypertension in the United States, 2003-2008. *Hypertension*, 2011, 57(6), 1076–80. doi, 10.1161 /HYPERTENSIONAHA.111.170308.

[17] Calhoun, DA; Jones, D; Textor, S; et al. Resistant hypertension, diagnosis, evaluation, and treatment, a scientific statement from the American Heart Association Professional Education Committee of the Council for High Blood Pressure Research. *Circulation*, 2008, 117(25), e510–26. doi, 10.1161/CIRCULATIONAHA.108.189141.

[18] Hamilton, W; Richards, D. In, Fisherman A, Richards D, eds. *Circulation of the Blood. Men and Ideas*, Bethesda, American Physiological Society, 1982, 87–90.
[19] Judy, WV; Watanabe, AM; Murphy, WR; Aprison, BS; Yu, PL. Sympathetic nerve activity and blood pressure in normotensive backcross rats genetically related to the spontaneously hypertensive rat. *Hypertension*, 1(6), 598–604. Available at, http, //www.ncbi.nlm.nih.gov/pubmed/541052. Accessed June 15, 2013.
[20] Winternitz, SR; Katholi, RE; Oparil, S. Role of the renal sympathetic nerves in the development and maintenance of hypertension in the spontaneously hypertensive rat. *The Journal of clinical investigation*, 1980, 66(5), 971–8. doi, 10.1172/JCI109966.
[21] Goldstein, DS. Plasma catecholamines and essential hypertension. An analytical review. *Hypertension*, 5(1), 86–99. Available at, http, //www.ncbi.nlm.nih.gov/pubmed/6336721. Accessed June 15, 2013.
[22] Grassi, G; Seravalle, G; Trevano, FQ; et al. Neurogenic abnormalities in masked hypertension. *Hypertension*, 2007, 50(3), 537–42. doi, 10.1161/HYPERTENSIONAHA,107.092528.
[23] Grassi, G; Seravalle, G; Quarti-Trevano, F; et al. Excessive sympathetic activation in heart failure with obesity and metabolic syndrome, characteristics and mechanisms. *Hypertension*, 2007, 49(3), 535–41. doi, 10.1161/01.HYP.0000255983.32896.b9.
[24] Grassi G; Seravalle G; Quarti-Trevano F; et al. Adrenergic, metabolic, and reflex abnormalities in reverse and extreme dipper hypertensives. *Hypertension*, 2008, 52(5), 925–31. doi, 10.1161/ HYPERTENSION AHA.108.116368.
[25] Grassi G. Assessment of sympathetic cardiovascular drive in human hypertension, achievements and perspectives. *Hypertension*. 2009, 54(4), 690–7. doi, 10.1161/HYPERTENSIONAHA.108.119883.
[26] Anderson, EA; Sinkey, CA; Lawton, WJ; Mark, AL. Elevated sympathetic nerve activity in borderline hypertensive humans. Evidence from direct intraneural recordings. *Hypertension*, 1989, 14(2), 177–83. Available at, http, //www.ncbi.nlm.nih.gov/pubmed/2759678. Accessed June 15, 2013.
[27] Grassi, G; Colombo, M; Seravalle, G; Spaziani, D; Mancia G. Dissociation between muscle and skin sympathetic nerve activity in essential hypertension, obesity, and congestive heart failure. *Hypertension*, 1998, 31(1), 64–7. Available at, http, //www.ncbi.nlm.nih.gov/pubmed/9449392. Accessed June 15, 2013.

[28] Grassi, G; Cattaneo, BM; Seravalle, G; Lanfranchi, A; Mancia, G. Baroreflex Control of Sympathetic Nerve Activity in Essential and Secondary Hypertension. *Hypertension*, 1998, 31(1), 68–72. doi, 10.1161/01.HYP.31.1.68.

[29] Grassi, G; Seravalle, G; Quarti-Trevano, F; et al. Adrenergic, metabolic, and reflex abnormalities in reverse and extreme dipper hypertensives. *Hypertension*. 2008, 52(5), 925–31. doi, 10.1161/ *Hypertensionaha*, 108.116368.

[30] Schlaich, MP; Lambert, E; Kaye, DM; et al. Sympathetic augmentation in hypertension, role of nerve firing, norepinephrine reuptake, and Angiotensin neuromodulation. *Hypertension*, 2004, 43(2), 169–75. doi, 10.1161/01.HYP.0000103160.35395.9E.

[31] Smith, PA; Graham, LN; Mackintosh, AF; Stoker, JB; Mary, DASG. Relationship between central sympathetic activity and stages of human hypertension. *American journal of hypertension*, 2004, 17(3), 217–22. doi, 10.1016/j.amjhyper.2003.10.010.

[32] Hogarth, AJ; Mackintosh, AF; Mary, DASG. The effect of gender on the sympathetic nerve hyperactivity of essential hypertension. *Journal of human hypertension*, 2007, 21(3), 239–45. doi, 10.1038/sj.jhh.1002132.

[33] Joyner, MJ; Charkoudian, N; Wallin, BG. A sympathetic view of the sympathetic nervous system and human blood pressure regulation. *Experimental physiology*, 2008, 93(6), 715–24. doi, 10.1113/expphysiol. 2007.039545.

[34] Esler, MD; Hasking, GJ; Willett, IR; Leonard, PW; Jennings, GL. Noradrenaline release and sympathetic nervous system activity. *Journal of hypertension*, 1985, 3(2), 117–29. Available at, http, //www.ncbi.nlm.nih.gov/pubmed/2991369. Accessed June 15, 2013.

[35] Esler, M; Jennings, G; Korner, P; et al. Assessment of human sympathetic nervous system activity from measurements of norepinephrine turnover. *Hypertension*, 1988, 11(1), 3–20. Available at, http, //www.ncbi.nlm.nih.gov/pubmed/2828236. Accessed June 15, 2013.

[36] Rumantir, MS; Vaz, M; Jennings, GL; et al. Neural mechanisms in human obesity-related hypertension. *Journal of hypertension*, 1999, 17(8), 1125–33. Available at, http, //www.ncbi.nlm.nih.gov/pubmed/ 10466468. Accessed June 15, 2013.

[37] Rumantir, MS; Kaye, DM; Jennings, GL; Vaz, M; Hastings, JA; Esler, MD. Phenotypic evidence of faulty neuronal norepinephrine reuptake in essential hypertension. *Hypertension*, 2000, 36(5), 824–9. Available at,

http, //www.ncbi.nlm.nih.gov/pubmed/11082150. Accessed June 15, 2013.

[38] Petersson, MJ; Rundqvist, B; Johansson, M; et al. Increased cardiac sympathetic drive in renovascular hypertension. *Journal of hypertension*, 2002, 20(6), 1181–7. Available at, http, //www.ncbi.nlm.nih.gov/pubmed/12023689. Accessed June 15, 2013.

[39] Esler, M; In, Zanchetti, A; Robertson, J; Birkenhager, W; eds. *Handbook of Hypertension*, vol. 22, *Hypertension Research in the Twentieth Century*. Amsterdam, Elsevier, 2004, 81–103.

[40] Kottke, FJ; Kubicek, WG; Visscher, MB. The production of arterial hypertension by chronic renal artery-nerve stimulation. *The American journal of physiology*, 1945, 145, 38–47. Available at, http, //www.ncbi.nlm.nih.gov/pubmed/21006702. Accessed June 15, 2013.

[41] Porlier, GA; Nadeau, RA; De Champlain, J; Bichet, DG. Increased circulating plasma catecholamines and plasma renin activity in dogs after chemical sympathectomy with 6-hydroxydopamine. *Canadian journal of physiology and pharmacology*, 1977, 55(3), 724–33. Available at, http, //www.ncbi.nlm.nih.gov/pubmed/884622. Accessed June 15, 2013.

[42] Crowley, SD; Gurley, SB; Herrera, MJ; et al. Angiotensin II causes hypertension and cardiac hypertrophy through its receptors in the kidney. *Proceedings of the National Academy of Sciences of the United States of America*, 2006, 103(47), 17985–90. doi, 10.1073/pnas. 0605545103.

[43] Salman, IM; Sattar, MA; Ameer, OZ; et al. Role of norepinephrine & angiotensin II in the neural control of renal sodium & water handling in spontaneously hypertensive rats. *The Indian journal of medical research*, 2010, 131, 786–92. Available at, http, //www.ncbi.nlm.nih.gov/pubmed /20571167. Accessed June 15, 2013.

[44] Hendel, MD; Collister, JP. Renal denervation attenuates long-term hypertensive effects of Angiotensin ii in the rat. *Clinical and experimental pharmacology & physiology*, 2006, 33(12), 1225–30. doi, 10.1111/j.1440-1681.2006.04514.x.

[45] Siddiqi, L; Joles, JA, Grassi, G; Blankestijn, PJ. Is kidney ischemia the central mechanism in parallel activation of the renin and sympathetic system? *Journal of hypertension*, 2009, 27(7), 1341–9. doi, 10.1097/HJH.0b013e32832b521b.

[46] Ye, S; Gamburd, M; Mozayeni, P; Koss, M; Campese, VM. A limited renal injury may cause a permanent form of neurogenic hypertension.

American journal of hypertension, 1998, 11(6 Pt 1), 723–8. Available at, http, //www.ncbi.nlm.nih.gov/pubmed/9657632. Accessed June 15, 2013.

[47] Converse, RL; Jacobsen, TN; Toto, RD; et al. Sympathetic overactivity in patients with chronic renal failure. *The New England journal of medicine*, 1992, 327(27), 1912–8. doi, 10.1056/ NEJM 1992123 13272 704.

[48] Hausberg, M; Kosch, M; Harmelink, P; et al. Sympathetic nerve activity in end-stage renal disease. *Circulation*, 2002, 106(15), 1974–9. Available at, http, //www.ncbi.nlm.nih.gov/pubmed/12370222. Accessed June 15, 2013.

[49] Wenting, GJ; Blankestijn, PJ; Poldermans, D; et al. Blood pressure response of nephrectomized subjects and patients with essential hypertension to ramipril, indirect evidence that inhibition of tissue angiotensin converting enzyme is important. *The American journal of cardiology*, 1987, 59(10), 92D–97D. Available at, http, //www.ncbi.nlm.nih.gov/pubmed/3034041. Accessed June 15, 2013.

[50] Klein, IHHT; Ligtenberg, G; Neumann, J; Oey, PL; Koomans, HA; Blankestijn, PJ. Sympathetic nerve activity is inappropriately increased in chronic renal disease. *Journal of the American Society of Nephrology, JASN*, 2003, 14(12), 3239–44. Available at, http, //www.ncbi.nlm.nih.gov/pubmed/14638922. Accessed June 15, 2013.

[51] Matsukawa, T; Gotoh, E; Minamisawa, K; et al. Effects of intravenous infusions of angiotensin II on muscle sympathetic nerve activity in humans. *The American journal of physiology*, 1991, 261(3 Pt 2), R690–6. Available at, http, //www.ncbi.nlm.nih.gov/pubmed/1887957. Accessed June 15, 2013.

[52] Kassab, S; Kato, T; Wilkins, FC; Chen, R; Hall, JE; Granger, JP. Renal denervation attenuates the sodium retention and hypertension associated with obesity. *Hypertension*, 1995, 25(4 Pt 2), 893–7. Available at, http, //www.ncbi.nlm.nih.gov/pubmed/7721450. Accessed June 15, 2013.

[53] Rippy, MK; Zarins, D; Barman, NC; Wu, A; Duncan, KL; Zarins, CK. Catheter-based renal sympathetic denervation, chronic preclinical evidence for renal artery safety. *Clinical research in cardiology, official journal of the German Cardiac Society*, 2011, 100(12), 1095–101. doi, 10.1007/s00392-011-0346-8.

[54] Rafiq, K; Noma, T; Fujisawa, Y. et al. Renal sympathetic denervation suppresses de novo podocyte injury and albuminuria in rats with aortic

regurgitation. *Circulation*. 2012, 125(11), 1402–13. doi, 10.1161/ *Circulationaha*,111.064097.

[55] Grimson, KS; Orgain, ES; Anderson, B; D'Angelo, GJ. Total thoracic and partial to total lumbar sympathectomy, splanchnicectomy and celiac ganglionectomy for hypertension. *Annals of surgery*, 1953, 138(4), 532–47. Available at, http, //www.pubmedcentral.nih.gov/ articlerender.fcgi?artid=1609434&tool=pmcentrez&rendertype=abstract. Accessed June 15, 2013.

[56] Peet, MM. Hypertension and its surgical treatment by bilateral supradiaphragmatic splanchnicectomy. *American journal of surgery*, 1948, 75(1), 48–68. Available at, http, //www.ncbi.nlm. nih.gov/pubmed/18918421. Accessed June 15, 2013.

[57] Smithwick, RH; Thompson, JE. Splanchnicectomy for essential hypertension, results in 1,266 cases. *Journal of the American Medical Association*, 1953, 152(16), 1501–4. Available at, http, //www.ncbi.nlm.nih.gov/pubmed/13061307. Accessed May 21, 2013.

[58] Schlaich, MP; Sobotka, PA; Krum, H; Lambert, E; Esler, MD. Renal sympathetic-nerve ablation for uncontrolled hypertension. *The New England journal of medicine*, 2009, 361(9), 932–4. doi, 10.1056/NEJMc0904179.

[59] Schlaich, MP; Sobotka, PA; Krum, H; Whitbourn, R; Walton, A; Esler, MD. Renal denervation as a therapeutic approach for hypertension, novel implications for an old concept. *Hypertension*. 2009, 54(6), 1195–201. doi, 10.1161/*Hypertensionaha*,109.138610.

[60] Krum, H; Schlaich, M; Whitbourn, R; et al. Catheter-based renal sympathetic denervation for resistant hypertension, a multicentre safety and proof-of-principle cohort study. *Lancet*, 2009, 373(9671), 1275–81. doi, 10.1016/S0140-6736(09)60566-3.

[61] Investigators, SH-1. Catheter-based renal sympathetic denervation for resistant hypertension, durability of blood pressure reduction out to 24 months. *Hypertension*. 2011, 57(5), 911–7. doi, 10.1161 /Hypertension aha,110.163014.

[62] Investigators, S-H; Esler, MD; Krum, H; et al. Renal sympathetic denervation in patients with treatment-resistant hypertension (The Symplicity HTN-2 Trial), a randomised controlled trial. *Lancet*, 2010, 376(9756), 1903–9. doi, 10.1016/S0140-6736(10)62039-9.

[63] Esler, MD; Krum, H; Schlaich, M; Schmieder, RE; Böhm, M; Sobotka, PA. Renal sympathetic denervation for treatment of drug-resistant hypertension, one-year results from the Symplicity HTN-2 randomized,

controlled trial. *Circulation*, 2012, 126(25), 2976–82. doi, 10.1161/*Circulationaha*,112.130880.

[64] Kandzari, DE; Bhatt, DL; Sobotka, PA; et al. Catheter-based renal denervation for resistant hypertension, rationale and design of the SYMPLICITY HTN-3 Trial. *Clinical cardiology*, 2012, 35(9), 528–35. doi, 10.1002/clc.22008.

[65] Chobanian, AV; Bakris, GL; Black, HR; et al. The Seventh Report of the Joint National Committee on Prevention, Detection, Evaluation, and Treatment of High Blood Pressure, the JNC 7 report. *JAMA, the journal of the American Medical Association*, 2003, 289(19), 2560–72. doi, 10.1001/jama.289.19.2560.

[66] Papademetriou, V; Doumas, M; Tsioufis, K. Renal Sympathetic Denervation for the Treatment of Difficult-to-Control or Resistant Hypertension. *International Journal of Hypertension*, 2011, 2011, 1–8. doi, 10.4061/2011/196518.

[67] Krum, H; Schlaich, M; Sobotka, P; Scheffers, I; Kroon, AA; De Leeuw, PW. Novel procedure- and device-based strategies in the management of systemic hypertension. *European heart journal*, 2011, 32(5), 537–44. doi, 10.1093/eurheartj/ehq457.

Index

A

acetylation, 40, 41
acetylcholine, 26, 58, 61
acetylcholinesterase, 59
acid, 3, 27, 48, 61
acidic, 3
active oxygen, 47
activity level, 53, 63, 64
AD, 25, 76
adaptability, 63
adaptation(s), 69, 99, 102
adenovirus, 128
adrenaline, 147
adulthood, 5
adults, 110, 151
advancements, 128
adverse effects, 148
aerobic capacity, 53, 64, 66, 67
aerobic exercise, 67, 95, 98, 119, 120, 121, 150
afferent nerve, 150
age, x, 17, 58, 64, 80, 81, 82, 99, 105, 109, 111, 112, 113, 119, 141, 142, 148, 151
aggregation, 130
albumin, 17
albuminuria, 146, 156
ALS, 28, 39, 43, 140
alters, 118, 150
American Heart Association, 151, 152

amino, 3, 9, 12, 50
amino acid(s), 3
ammonia, 140
amplitude, 118
amygdala, 5, 63
amyotrophic lateral sclerosis, 37, 39, 41, 43
anatomy, vii, 150
androgen, 131
anemia, viii, 2, 3, 16, 17, 18, 22, 29, 34, 35, 36, 41, 43, 44, 46
angiogenesis, 6, 19, 31, 41, 44
angioplasty, 67
angiotensin converting enzyme, 156
angiotensin II, 145, 146, 152, 155, 156
angiotensin II receptor antagonist, 152
anhidrosis, 61, 146
anoxia, 24
ANS, viii, ix, 52, 58, 60, 62, 67, 79, 80, 81, 83, 84, 86, 93, 94, 95, 101, 103, 104, 105, 106, 107, 113, 114
anthropometric characteristics, 84
antibody, 24, 25, 27, 61
antigen, 64
antioxidant, 127
aortic regurgitation, 146, 157
aplasia, 32
aplastic anemia, 2
apoptosis, 10, 11, 12, 13, 14, 16, 19, 20, 21, 22, 23, 24, 25, 26, 27, 28, 30, 32, 38, 41,

42, 45, 46, 47, 49, 50, 126, 130, 131, 135, 136, 137, 138, 139
apoptotic pathways, 34
appetite, 16
arginine, 3
arrhythmias, 62, 102
arterial hypertension, 152, 155
arteriogram, 147
arteritis, 53
artery(s), 20, 21, 43, 53, 57, 102, 131, 132, 144, 145, 147, 148, 150, 155, 156
arthritis, 53, 59
aryl hydrocarbon receptor, 6
asparagines, 4
aspartate, 35
assessment, vii, ix, 60, 64, 91, 93, 101, 103
astrocytes, 5, 7, 8, 23, 24, 25, 30, 32, 42
asymmetry, 27, 33
asymptomatic, 142
atelectasis, 146
atherosclerosis, viii, ix, 52, 53, 54, 57, 123, 128, 131, 139, 140
atherosclerotic plaque, 131, 139
athletes, 81, 96, 97, 103, 108, 109, 112, 115, 116, 118, 119, 120
atrial fibrillation, 102, 115
atrophy, 26
attitudes, 64
automaticity, 60
autonomic activity, 117, 120
autonomic function, vii, viii, 52, 67, 69, 70, 97, 113, 115, 119, 120
autonomic nervous system, viii, 52, 79, 80, 87, 95, 98, 99, 102, 103, 112, 117, 118, 119, 121
autonomic neuropathy, 60
aversion, 59
awareness, 151
axonal degeneration, 28

basal lamina, 18
basal metabolic rate, 82
basement membrane, 19
beneficial effect, 20, 22, 23, 66, 90, 92
benefits, 80, 102, 142
benign, 131
bioavailability, 8
biochemistry, 133, 134
biological activities, 29
biological activity, vii, 1, 3, 4, 24
biosynthesis, 35
bleeding, 22
bleeding time, 22
blood, vii, 2, 4, 17, 18, 19, 21, 23, 29, 39, 43, 46, 53, 56, 60, 61, 65, 92, 94, 103, 113, 116, 117, 120, 142, 143, 145, 146, 147, 148, 149, 150, 151, 153, 154, 157
blood circulation, 18
blood flow, 21, 23, 145
blood pressure, 18, 39, 56, 60, 61, 65, 92, 94, 103, 113, 116, 117, 120, 142, 143, 145, 146, 147, 148, 149, 150, 151, 153, 154, 157
blood pressure reduction, 142, 146, 148, 149, 157
blood supply, 19
blood vessels, vii, 19, 53, 143
body mass index (BMI), viii, 52, 55, 64, 65, 81, 84, 113
body weight, 8
bonds, 4, 125
bone, 4, 16, 19, 31, 49, 53
bone marrow, 4, 16, 19, 31, 49
bradycardia, 89, 97, 98, 99, 106, 112
brain, 5, 7, 12, 15, 19, 23, 25, 27, 30, 32, 33, 35, 42, 49, 59, 63, 120, 126, 135
brainstem, 63
branching, 19
breathing, 44, 120
breathlessness, 22, 146

B

back pain, 148
backcross, 153
Bangladesh, 73

C

Ca^{2+}, 124, 125, 129, 131
caffeine, 82

Index

calcium, ix, 15, 18, 123
caliber, 143
calorie, 150
cancer, 50
capillary, 18, 19, 21, 49
carbohydrate(s), 3, 4, 47
carboxyl, 9
cardiac arrhythmia, 60
cardiac autonomic function, vii, 69, 70
cardiac involvement, viii, 52, 53
cardiac output, 22
cardiomyopathy, x, 30, 129, 137
cardiovascular disease(s), vii, viii, x, 2, 47, 52, 54, 65, 66, 67, 113, 124, 128, 131, 133, 134, 152
cardiovascular disorders, ix, 95, 102
cardiovascular function, 61, 80, 102
cardiovascular risk, viii, 52, 54, 55
cardiovascular system, vii, ix, 117, 123
carpal tunnel syndrome, 57
cartilage, 53
cascades, 33, 35
caspases, 16
catecholamines, 61, 153, 155
catheter, 146, 147
CBP, 6, 7
cDNA, 38, 45
cell biology, 134, 136, 139
cell death, x, 12, 19, 27, 46, 123, 124, 126, 128, 129, 130, 135, 140
cell differentiation, 15
cell division, 15
cell line, 26
cell signaling, vii, 2, 16, 29
cell surface, 48
central nervous system (CNS), 5, 6, 14, 23, 28, 29, 30, 143, 145
ceramide, 138
cerebral blood flow, 19, 41, 63
cerebrospinal fluid, 5, 28, 39
chaperones, x, 123, 125, 128, 129, 133, 137, 139
chemical, 48, 133, 143, 155
chemical properties, 48
CHF, 111

Chicago, 2
children, 97, 112, 119
China, 1
cholesterol, 64, 113, 131, 139
choline, 26
chromosome, 3, 13, 36
chronic heart failure, 23, 109, 112, 115, 120, 142
chronic hypoxia, 32
chronic kidney disease, 17, 35, 46
chronic renal failure, 16, 36, 46, 156
circulation, vii, 16
civil servants, 98
CKD, 145, 149
classes, 143, 152
cleavage, 3, 45, 130
clinical application, 3
clinical interventions, 80
clinical trials, 143
clonus, 27
cognition, 15
cognitive dysfunction, 46
cognitive function, 25
collagen, 146
community, 66, 151
complex interactions, 53, 54
complexity, 114
compliance, 149
complications, 29, 50, 69, 146, 147
compounds, 124
conditioning, 110, 112
conduction, 53, 60, 129
conflict, 105
congenital heart disease, 128
congestive heart failure, 22, 46, 153
Congress, 148
congruence, 145
constipation, 61
construction, 9
control group, 62, 67, 69, 148
controlled trials, 36
controversial, 80, 114
controversies, 113
COPD, 96, 108, 110, 119, 120
coronary artery bypass graft, 67

coronary artery disease, 95, 102, 111, 139
coronary heart disease, 29, 65, 80, 95, 110, 121
correlation, 114, 132
cortex, 4, 5, 7, 25, 26
cortical neurons, 5, 9, 43, 45
cost, 16, 17, 149, 150
counseling, 152
cross sectional study, 107, 108, 109, 110, 111
cross-sectional study, 90
CRP, viii, 52, 57, 59, 60
culture, 28, 32, 130
culture media, 130
cure, 63
CV, viii, 51, 52, 53, 54, 55, 56, 57, 58, 63, 64, 66, 69, 70, 111
CVD, 52, 65
cycling, 117
cysteine, 15, 33
cytochrome, 14, 33
cytokines, 9, 28, 40, 58, 62
cytoplasm, 13
cytoprotectant, 23
cytotoxicity, 135, 139

D

daily living, 66
danger, 63
data set, 82, 83, 84
DBP, 147
deaths, 142
decay, 129
deductive reasoning, viii, 80
defects, 53
deficiency, 16, 32
degradation, x, 3, 6, 7, 13, 15, 26, 38, 123, 128, 136
dementia, 142
demyelinating disease, 28
demyelination, 28, 37
Department of Health and Human Services, 115
dephosphorylation, 15, 132

depolarization, 14, 45
deprivation, 23
derivatives, 28, 29, 45
destruction, 38, 53, 66
developing brain, 35, 46
deviation, 68, 82, 86, 89, 111
diabetes, 17, 32, 42, 50, 55, 60, 124, 148
diabetic patients, 98, 110, 120
dialysis, 16, 17, 27, 39, 41, 121
diastolic blood pressure, 62, 142
diastolic pressure, 21
diet, 81, 113, 142
dihydroxyphenylalanine, 24, 26, 61
dilated cardiomyopathy, x, 123, 129, 137
dilation, 128
dimerization, 12, 125
dioxin, 38
disease activity, 64, 66
disease model, 39
diseases, vii, viii, 2, 29, 53, 60, 61, 69, 124, 144, 149, 150
disorder, 26, 59, 61
dissociation, 10, 14
distribution, 8, 9, 83, 84, 85, 89
diuretic, 143, 147
DNA, 3, 10, 11, 12, 13, 24, 41, 134
DNA damage, 10, 13
dogs, 37, 139, 145, 146, 155
domain structure, 9
dominance, 111
donors, 24
dopamine, 39
dopaminergic, 26, 46, 49
dosage, 16, 18, 22
dosing, 16, 21, 142
down-regulation, 25, 48
drug discovery, 44
drug targets, 133
drugs, 147
dry eyes, 61
durability, 157
dysplasia, 102

Index

E

EAE, 28, 49
ECs, 5, 18, 19, 23, 24
editors, 70
effluents, 145
effusion, 53
ejaculation, 146
electrolyte, 147
electron, 138
elongation, 140
elucidation, 23
embryogenesis, 5
encephalomyelitis, 45
encoding, 3, 127
end stage renal disease, 17
endocardium, 53
endothelial cells (ECs), 4, 7, 30, 44, 47, 48, 49, 131, 139
endothelium, 104, 149
end-stage renal disease, 16, 17, 31, 36, 43, 156
endurance, 67, 92, 96, 97, 98, 99, 102, 103, 105, 106, 112, 113, 115, 116, 117, 119, 120, 122
energy, viii, 16, 63, 79, 82, 124
energy consumption, 82
energy expenditure, viii, 63, 79, 82
enlargement, 60
environment(s), 35, 64, 81, 88, 125
environmental change, 125
enzyme(s), 40, 125
EPC, 19
ependymal, 7
ependymal cell, 7
epilepsy, 27, 62
epileptogenesis, 39
episcleritis, 57
epithelial cells, 8, 44, 50
erythrocyte sedimentation rate, 57, 66
erythrocytes, 16
erythrocytosis, 31
erythroid cells, vii, 1, 42
erythropoietin, vii, 1, 2, 7, 30, 31, 32, 33, 34, 35, 36, 37, 38, 39, 40, 41, 42, 43, 44, 45, 46, 47, 48, 49, 50
ESR, 57, 66
ESRD, 142, 144
estrogen, 8, 42
ethnicity, 81
etiology, x, 142, 143
eukaryotic, 10, 13, 126, 140
evidence, viii, x, 4, 52, 53, 57, 61, 63, 64, 80, 84, 106, 142, 143, 144, 145, 147, 154, 156
excitation, 103, 124
exclusion, 147
exercise performance, 115
exercise programs, viii, 80, 88, 103
exertion, 102, 115
experimental autoimmune encephalomyelitis, 28, 30
exposure, 16, 19, 24, 25, 150

F

fear, 66
febrile seizure, 27, 39
fetus, 49
fiber(s), 59, 60, 144, 145, 149
fibrinogen, 64
fibroblasts, 4, 44
fibromyalgia, 121
fibrosis, 20
financial, 142
Finland, 82
Fisherman, 153
fitness, 64, 65, 95, 98, 105, 106, 111, 112, 113, 115, 118, 119
flexibility, 57, 67
fluctuations, 63
fluid, 145, 150
football, 121
Ford, 76, 119
forebrain, 46
formation, 18, 25, 27, 40, 49, 61, 125, 131
France, 2
free radicals, 41

Index

G

ganglion, 50, 116
gastroparesis, 61
gene expression, 4, 36, 42, 43, 45, 124, 126
gene regulation, 31
gene silencing, 13, 16
genes, 6, 10, 11, 12, 13, 15, 22, 126, 127, 128, 130, 136
genetics, 137, 140
geometry, 69
glaucoma, 50
glial cells, 23
glucose, 16, 23, 24, 34, 38, 125, 134, 139
glutamate, 4, 24, 28, 43
glycans, 47
glycine, 4
glycogen, 10, 11, 33, 41
glycosylation, 3
growth, vii, 1, 10, 13, 15, 19, 23, 34, 50, 129, 131
growth arrest, 10, 13
growth factor, vii, 1, 23
growth signal, 50
GTPases, 131

H

half-life, 8, 9
headache, 17
healing, x, 37, 124
healing potential, x, 124
health, 17, 53, 63, 65, 67, 69, 70, 80, 90, 110, 115, 124, 133, 142
health care, 142
health problems, 124
heart disease, 19, 23, 128, 130, 131, 152
heart failure, x, 22, 23, 47, 55, 123, 124, 128, 129, 131, 133, 139, 149, 153
heart rate (HR), vii, viii, 52, 58, 62, 63, 68, 69, 70, 80, 82, 83, 86, 88, 89, 90, 91, 92, 94, 96, 97, 98, 99, 103, 110, 115, 116, 117, 119, 120, 121
heart rate variability (HRV), vii, viii, 52, 80

hematocrit, 16, 17, 18
hematopoietic growth, vii, 1, 23
hemodialysis, 17, 34, 40, 41, 45, 46, 110
hemoglobin, 5, 8, 17, 35
hepatocytes, 4
heterogeneity, 80
high blood pressure, 18, 56, 144
hippocampus, 5, 25, 26, 27
history, 55, 81
HIV, 107, 118
HLA, 57
HM, 11
homeostasis, ix, 64, 123, 125, 129, 131, 133, 139, 143, 147, 150
homocysteine, 64
hormone, 2
hospitalization, 22, 148
human, vii, 1, 2, 3, 5, 6, 8, 15, 16, 18, 19, 21, 22, 23, 26, 27, 30, 31, 34, 36, 37, 38, 39, 41, 42, 43, 44, 45, 46, 47, 48, 124, 129, 132, 143, 146, 147, 153, 154
human body, vii, 1
human brain, 5, 39
human leukemia cells, 15
Hunter, 74, 137
hyperactivity, 154
hypertension, vii, viii, ix, x, 18, 27, 29, 45, 52, 55, 56, 96, 102, 115, 121, 122, 123, 128, 131, 141, 142, 143, 144, 145, 146, 149, 150, 151, 152, 153, 154, 155, 156, 157, 158
hypertrophy, ix, 22, 60, 102, 123, 128, 129, 131, 136, 144, 155
hypotension, 148
hypothesis, 2, 4, 143, 145
hypoxia, 2, 4, 5, 6, 7, 8, 23, 24, 26, 27, 31, 32, 36, 38, 39, 40, 42, 47, 48, 105, 126, 128, 129, 130
hypoxia-inducible factor, 5, 7, 32, 38, 40, 48

I

identification, 4, 61, 103
idiopathic, 60, 61
IFN, 28

Index

immune function, 58
immune system, 62
immunization, 28
immunomodulatory, 62
immunoreactivity, 4, 47
impairments, 53
improvements, 27, 88, 142
in vitro, 20, 31, 41, 43, 46, 62
in vivo, 20, 22, 34, 35, 44, 46, 62, 131, 139, 140
incidence, 17, 29, 55, 80, 102
individual differences, 113
individuals, viii, x, 52, 65, 70, 92, 102, 113, 141, 142
inducer, 132, 139
induction, x, 6, 8, 11, 13, 14, 15, 28, 40, 43, 44, 46, 123, 128, 130, 132, 134, 136, 137
inertia, 142
infarction, 102
infection, 59, 81
inflammation, viii, 28, 34, 39, 52, 53, 54, 57, 58, 59, 63, 66
inflammatory arthritis, 59
inflammatory disease, viii, 51, 53, 58
inflammatory responses, 27
informed consent, 81, 82
inhibition, 15, 20, 59, 126, 130, 136, 156
inhibitor, 48, 64, 128, 132, 140
initiation, 10, 13, 125, 126
injury(s), 9, 11, 14, 15, 20, 24, 25, 26, 32, 33, 34, 39, 41, 45, 47, 130, 136, 137, 138, 146, 149, 155, 156
inositol, 125
insecurity, 63
insulin, 4, 42, 149
insulin resistance, 149
integration, 41, 50, 63, 136
integrity, 3, 15, 23, 24, 32, 33, 34, 41, 45
interference, 13, 48
interneurons, 25
intervention, viii, ix, 23, 43, 52, 64, 67, 69, 70, 80, 81, 82, 84, 85, 86, 88, 89, 90, 92, 93, 94, 95, 107, 108, 109, 110, 111, 112, 121, 140, 149
intervention response, 93

intracellular calcium, 18
intravenously, 21
intron, 126
invertebrates, 137
Iowa, 97
iron, 18, 22, 46
ischemia, ix, 19, 20, 21, 22, 24, 31, 34, 36, 41, 48, 123, 128, 130, 137, 138, 145, 155
ischemia-reperfusion injury, 20, 22, 31, 48
isolation, 60
issues, 133

J

Japan, 2, 65
joint damage, 64
joint destruction, 66
joint pain, 66, 69
joints, viii, 51, 53, 63, 66, 67
Jordan, 77, 99

K

kidney(s), x, 2, 4, 6, 8, 17, 32, 35, 36, 38, 46, 47, 142, 143, 144, 145, 146, 147, 149, 150, 155
kinase activity, 48

L

lack of control, 147
latency, 27
lateral sclerosis, 28, 140
lead, x, 8, 12, 18, 22, 25, 29, 69, 88, 113, 123, 131, 145
left ventricle, 21
lesions, 132, 146
leucine, 128, 134
liberation, 11
lice, 32
life expectancy, 65
ligand, 9, 22, 49
light, x, 34, 106, 118, 142
lipids, 124

lithium, 27, 46
liver, 2, 4, 6, 40, 135, 140
liver cancer, 40
localization, 36, 39
longevity, 42
low-density lipoprotein, 64
lumen, 125, 126, 127
lung cancer, 110, 121
Luo, 32
lymphocytes, 28
lymphoma, 128

M

Mackintosh, 154
macrophages, 58, 131, 139
magnitude, 91, 104, 144, 148
majority, 91, 114
malignancy, 16, 41
mammalian cells, 6
man, 98
management, 26, 34, 53, 56, 58, 60, 62, 66, 146, 151, 152, 158
marrow, 19
mass, viii, 18, 39, 52, 55, 65, 81, 84
matrix, 19
MB, 155
MBP, 28
measurement(s), ix, x, 80, 81, 82, 88, 91, 93, 95, 97, 101, 103, 104, 105, 106, 114, 116, 141, 154
mechanical stress, 140
median, 147
medical, 61, 81, 155
medication, 17, 81
medicine, 93, 134, 135, 137, 139, 140, 152, 156, 157
mellitus, 69
memory, 26
menstruation, 19
mesenchymal stem cells, 16, 26, 35
meta-analysis, 23, 36, 53, 63, 88, 104, 151
metabolic syndrome, 149, 153
metabolism, 4, 124, 140
metalloproteinase, 48

methodology, 64, 143
mice, 20, 25, 26, 28, 32, 36, 37, 40, 41, 46, 47, 49, 50, 126, 128, 129, 130, 135, 137, 140
microRNA, 130
midbrain, 5
migration, 18, 19, 25, 48
miniature, 151
mitochondria, 14, 124
mitogen, vii, 1, 12, 42
model system, 31
models, 58, 139, 146
modifications, 106, 111, 142
molecular structure, 2
molecular weight, 3
molecules, x, 4, 124
Moon, 20, 21, 22, 42, 43
morbidity, x, 60, 62, 69, 70, 80, 141, 146
morphology, 150
mortality, x, 27, 53, 69, 80, 95, 102, 115, 128, 141, 142, 146, 151
mortality rate, 27, 128
mortality risk, 53, 142
motif, 9, 11
motor neuron disease, 28
motor neurons, 28, 29
mRNA, 5, 8, 19, 30, 34, 49, 126, 127, 129, 146
muscle atrophy, 28, 53
muscle contraction, 53, 98, 116
muscle strength, 64, 66, 67
muscles, 145
mutant, 129, 137
myelin, 5, 28, 32
myelin basic protein, 28
myelin oligodendrocyte glycoprotein, 28
myocardial infarction, 20, 21, 30, 31, 32, 36, 37, 42, 43, 47, 49, 67, 102, 115, 128
myocardial ischemia, 20
myocarditis, 53
myocardium, 19, 20, 21, 31, 37, 53
myocyte, 21, 130, 137
myosin, 21

N

National Academy of Sciences, 135, 138, 155
necrosis, 20
negative consequences, 102
neovascularization, 23, 37, 44, 47
nerve, 58, 61, 62, 117, 143, 145, 147, 153, 154, 155, 156, 157
nerve fibers, 59
nervous system, 5, 13, 15, 29, 33, 37, 91, 99, 103, 111, 117, 150
neuroblastoma, 6, 23
neurodegeneration, 15
neurodegenerative diseases, vii, 2, 25, 34, 124, 126, 135
neurodegenerative disorders, 140
neurofibrillary tangles, 25
neurogenesis, 25, 26, 37, 39, 40
neuroimaging, 61, 63
neurological disability, 28
neuronal apoptosis, 23, 24
neuronal cells, 5, 14, 32
neuronal stem cells, 25
neurons, 5, 7, 8, 13, 23, 24, 25, 26, 39, 42, 49, 58, 139
neuropathy, 60
neuroprotection, 12, 25, 33, 34, 35, 37, 39, 41, 45
neurotoxicity, 12, 16, 24, 27, 35, 44
neurotransmitter(s), 58, 59
New England, 139, 152, 156, 157
NH_2, 14, 139
nicotinamide, 42
nitric oxide, 24, 42
nodules, 57
norepinephrine, 18, 37, 58, 61, 147, 150, 154, 155
normal aging, 112
normal distribution, 84
North America, 97, 116
Norway, 65
nucleus, 6, 7, 11, 12, 13, 15, 16, 124, 126
null, 25
nutrient(s), 130, 134

O

obesity, 65, 122, 124, 146, 149, 153, 154, 156
occlusion, 20, 21
old age, 111
oligodendrocytes, 24
oligosaccharide, 3
opportunities, 134
organ(s), 4, 40, 53, 56, 122, 144
organelle(s), ix, 123, 124, 125
orthostatic hypotension, 146
orthostatic intolerance, 61
oscillation, 56, 119
osteoarthritis, 59
osteoclastogenesis, 49
overtraining, ix, 101, 114
oviduct, 4, 42
ox, vii
oxidation, 41, 140
oxidative stress, ix, 13, 19, 24, 33, 123, 125
oxygen, 3, 4, 5, 6, 7, 17, 23, 30, 31, 32, 42, 44, 69, 130
oxygen consumption, 23, 69

P

p53, 26, 40
pain, 63, 66, 76
palpitations, 146
pannus formation, 53
parallel, 59, 145, 155
parasympathetic activity, 63, 92, 103, 120
parasympathetic nervous system, 62, 111, 143
participants, viii, 79, 81, 82, 88, 89, 106, 109, 143
pathogenesis, x, 122, 141, 149, 150
pathology, 124, 129
pathophysiological, 26, 143
pathophysiology, 128, 145, 147, 149
pathways, vii, viii, x, 1, 2, 9, 10, 12, 15, 16, 29, 32, 33, 52, 58, 63, 123, 124, 139
peptide, 3, 21, 25, 28, 57, 120, 126, 135

perfusion, 19, 30, 31
pericarditis, 53, 57
pericardium, 53
peripheral blood, 22, 62
peripheral blood mononuclear cell, 22
permission, 54, 55, 56, 65
peroxide, 32
pharmaceutical(s), 3, 133, 150
pharmacokinetics, 31, 140
pharmacology, 36, 136, 155
phenol, 145
phenotype(s), 26, 44, 129
Philadelphia, 70, 71, 73, 76
phosphate, 11, 34
phospholipids, ix, 41, 123, 125
phosphorylation, 9, 10, 11, 12, 14, 15, 16, 36, 40, 44, 47, 50, 127, 131, 132
physical activity, viii, 52, 63, 64, 65, 66, 70, 80, 98, 102, 111, 119, 120
physical exercise, 65, 66, 96, 119
Physiological, 97, 153
physiological mechanisms, 147
physiology, vii, 36, 45, 93, 116, 136, 138, 154, 155, 156
PI3K, 9, 10, 11, 16, 22, 26, 29, 41, 45, 126, 135, 139
placebo, 36
placenta, 4
plaque, 26, 132
plasma levels, 58, 61, 144
plasma membrane, 9, 11, 125
plasminogen, 64
playing, x, 141
plexus, 144
PM, 139, 151
Poincaré, viii, 80, 81, 82, 97, 104, 114
polarity, 15
polyamine, 50
polymerase, 5
polymerase chain reaction, 5
polypeptide(s), 3, 125
population, ix, 53, 63, 64, 66, 88, 101, 103, 111
precursor cells, 24
prefrontal cortex, 63

pregnancy, 144
preservation, 69
prevention, viii, 20, 24, 52, 65, 66, 70, 80, 152
probe, 98, 116
profit, 3
progenitor cells, 16, 25, 28, 41, 48
progesterone, 8
prognosis, 113
programming, 146
pro-inflammatory, 22, 58
proliferation, 13, 18, 19, 20, 22, 23, 25, 27, 28, 32, 36, 45, 53
proline, 4, 10, 38
promoter, 12, 126, 128, 129, 130
proteasome, 6, 38, 127, 128, 132, 140
protection, 9, 12, 13, 16, 20, 22, 24, 25, 33, 41, 47, 82, 137
protein family, 13, 128
protein kinase C, 11
protein kinases, vii, 1, 12, 135
protein synthesis, ix, 123, 125, 129
protein tyrosine phosphatases, vii, 1, 9
proteins, x, 9, 11, 12, 13, 15, 44, 123, 124, 125, 127, 128, 129, 131, 134, 137
proto-oncogene, 15
psychological processes, ix, 101, 114
public awareness, 142
pulmonary circulation, vii
PUMA, 26, 40, 130, 138
purification, 2
P-value, 84, 85, 86, 89

Q

QRS complex, 62, 68
QT interval, 59
quality control, 125, 134, 136, 137
quality of life, 17, 64
quantification, 81, 83, 93, 104, 114

R

radiation, 150

radicals, 47
rapamycin, vii, 1, 9, 10, 11, 14, 34
rat kidneys, 39
RE, 139, 153, 157
reactive oxygen, 41, 125
reactivity, 112, 140
reading, 96
receptors, 9, 47, 48, 62, 145, 155
recognition, 6, 26, 56
recombinant DNA, 48
recommendations, viii, ix, 52, 95, 102
recovery, 20, 49, 105, 117, 130
recycling, 129
red blood cells, 2, 5, 29
redistribution, ix, 80, 94
regeneration, 31
regression, 108
rehabilitation, 66, 67, 95, 108, 110, 111, 112, 115, 121
rehabilitation program, 95, 108, 112
relevance, 22, 134, 151
remediation, 129
remodelling, 96, 122, 138
remyelination, 28
renal failure, 3, 18, 37
renin, 46, 145, 147, 155
repair, 19, 32
repellent, 59
repression, 128
reproductive organs, 4, 8
researchers, 62, 114
residues, 3, 11, 12, 37
resistance, 18, 29, 50, 64, 105, 110, 112, 113, 117, 118, 121, 135
resources, 33
respiration, 60, 103
responsiveness, 16, 18, 37, 81, 90, 93
restoration, 41
reticulum, vii, ix, 123, 124, 129, 133, 134, 135, 136, 137, 138, 139, 140
retina, 23
RH, 140, 157
rheology, 45
rheumatic diseases, 65, 66
rheumatoid arthritis, vii, 54, 55, 63, 66

rheumatoid factor, 57
right ventricle, 102
rings, 19
risk, viii, 17, 21, 23, 52, 53, 54, 55, 56, 57, 59, 62, 63, 64, 65, 66, 67, 69, 70, 102, 131, 142
risk factors, viii, 52, 53, 54, 55, 56, 57, 65, 66, 70, 102
risk profile, 64
RNA, 13, 48
rodents, 5, 31
root, 84, 86, 89

S

safety, 36, 63, 140, 146, 149, 150, 156, 157
SAP, 109, 111
saturation, 17
scaling, 114
scatter, 104
sclerosis, 28
secrete, 4
secretion, 3, 17, 35, 129, 145
seizure, 27, 40, 42
self-control, 81
sensing, 30, 38, 134
sensitivity, viii, 52, 61, 97, 104, 106, 118, 119, 121
sensor proteins, 125
sepsis, 135
serine, 4, 11, 13, 24, 125, 126
serum, 2, 8, 17, 19, 21, 31, 37, 39, 40, 43, 60
serum albumin, 17
serum EPO, 8, 21
serum erythropoietin, 43
sex, 64, 82
shear, 131, 139
sheep, 2
showing, 103
sialic acid, 3, 4
side chain, 3
signal transduction, vii, x, 1, 9, 10, 15, 29, 33, 123, 125

signaling pathway, x, 15, 26, 33, 41, 44, 49, 124, 131, 139
signalling, 35
signals, 9, 11, 39, 58, 125, 140
signs, 104, 112
sinus arrhythmia, 103
skeletal muscle, 144
skin, 144, 153
sleep apnea, 149
smoking, viii, 52, 55, 64
smooth muscle, 4, 18, 30, 131, 149
smooth muscle cells, 131, 149
SNS, 105, 107, 108, 109, 111
society, 142
sodium, 140, 145, 146, 150, 155, 156
software, 82
South Africa, viii, 51, 52, 79, 101
species, 41, 125
spectral component, 106
sphincter, 60
spinal cord, 28, 32, 49
spinal cord injury, 49
spleen, 4
stability, 32, 67, 111
standard deviation, 68, 82, 84, 86, 88, 89, 106
standardization, 114
starvation, 125, 130
state(s), ix, 9, 30, 62, 67, 81, 92, 93, 117, 123, 125, 126, 133, 136, 138, 144
statistics, 64, 104, 151
status epilepticus, 27, 46
stem cells, 46
stent, 23
steroids, ix, 123, 124, 125
stimulation, 12, 15, 42, 48, 58, 62, 67, 90, 93, 96, 143, 145, 155
stimulus, 58, 81, 93, 145
storage, 124, 125
strength training, 67
stress, vii, ix, 24, 34, 45, 62, 95, 123, 124, 125, 126, 127, 128, 129, 130, 131, 132, 133, 134, 135, 136, 137, 138, 139, 140, 147

stress response, 126, 128, 130, 134, 136, 137, 147
stretching, 67
striatum, 25, 26, 27
stroke, 22, 25, 34, 37, 65, 131, 142, 151
stroke volume, 22
stromal cells, 19, 49
structural changes, 102
structure, 3, 45, 63
subcutaneous injection, 8
subgroups, 148
substrate(s), 10, 12, 14, 33, 41, 48, 136
Sun, 26, 47, 49, 135
suppression, 13, 40, 105, 130
survival, 9, 11, 13, 16, 20, 23, 24, 25, 27, 29, 31, 32, 33, 35, 49, 50, 58, 69
susceptibility, 42, 96, 120, 122
sympathectomy, 143, 155, 157
sympathetic denervation, vii, x, 141, 146, 156, 157
sympathetic fibers, 145
sympathetic nerve fibers, 59, 143
sympathetic nervous system, x, 58, 62, 88, 91, 105, 112, 141, 149, 150, 154
sympathetic variation, ix, 80
symptoms, 16, 26, 28, 60, 61, 63, 102
syndrome, 57, 139, 146
synovial tissue, 58
synthesis, ix, 123, 124, 125
systolic blood pressure, 64, 103, 108

T

T cell, 15
tachycardia, 146
tamoxifen, 137
target, vii, x, 1, 9, 10, 11, 13, 14, 17, 33, 34, 48, 56, 124, 127, 128, 130, 132, 141
Task Force, 97, 113, 116, 152
tau, 25, 47
techniques, viii, x, 68, 80, 81, 82, 91, 113, 114, 141
tendons, 53
tension, 4, 5
terminals, 59, 145

Index

testing, 82
testis, 4
textbook, 71
therapeutic agents, 132
therapeutic benefits, 21
therapeutic interventions, x, 124, 133
therapeutic targets, 135
therapeutics, 152
therapy, 9, 17, 18, 21, 22, 23, 24, 30, 31, 32, 39, 40, 43, 46, 50, 62, 66, 88, 95, 96, 113, 115, 121, 128, 142, 148, 152
thermal stability, 3
thermoregulation, 60, 104
threonine, 11, 13, 125, 126
thrombosis, 23, 27, 139
time periods, 91
time series, 114
tissue, 5, 6, 8, 19, 34, 36, 40, 53, 59, 60, 64, 128, 129, 156
TNF, 13, 23, 28, 126
tonometry, 57
total energy, 63
toxicity, 13, 16, 24, 26, 33
TP53, 22
trafficking, 34
training, vii, viii, ix, 64, 67, 69, 79, 80, 81, 82, 84, 88, 92, 95, 96, 97, 98, 99, 101, 102, 103, 106, 107, 108, 109, 110, 111, 112, 113, 114, 115, 116, 118, 119, 120, 121, 122, 150
training programs, 113
transcription, vii, 1, 5, 6, 7, 10, 11, 12, 13, 31, 41, 44, 45, 125, 126, 127, 128, 129, 131, 134, 135
transcription factors, 12, 41, 129, 134
transducer, vii, 1, 9, 10, 44, 128
transduction, 9, 15
transfection, 9, 14
transferrin, 17
transformation, 84
transfusion, 16, 17
translation, x, 123, 126, 127, 135
translocation, 10, 13, 16, 33, 126, 128, 135
transplantation, 19, 26
transport, 17

treatment, 3, 8, 16, 17, 18, 20, 21, 22, 23, 24, 31, 36, 41, 49, 62, 66, 124, 128, 142, 148, 151, 152, 157
tremor, 26
trial, 3, 36, 43, 115, 147, 148, 149, 157, 158
triggers, 16, 124, 128, 130, 131, 133, 136
tumor, 15, 19, 23, 126
tumor growth, 19
tumor necrosis factor, 23, 126
tumorigenesis, 37
turnover, 143, 154
type 2 diabetes, 67, 69, 118, 139
tyrosine, vii, 1, 9, 10, 11, 12, 34, 36, 37, 44, 48, 49

U

ubiquitin, 6, 13, 38, 136
ubiquitin-proteasome system, 136
unfolded protein response (UPR), ix, 123, 124
United States (USA), x, 65, 135, 138, 141, 142, 151, 152, 155
urea, 17, 140
urea cycle, 140
urinary retention, 61
urinary tract infection, 148
urine, 2
US Department of Health and Human Services, 115
uterus, 4, 8, 32

V

vagus nerve, 58, 62, 63
variables, 67, 68, 69, 70, 84
variations, 149
vascular endothelial growth factor (VEGF), 19
vascular system, 29
vasculature, 131
vasculitis, 57
vasoconstriction, 143, 145
vasodilation, 44, 143

vasodilator, 120
vasomotor, 104, 143
vasomotor nerves, 143
vector, 27
velocity, 56
ventilation, 115
ventricle, 21
ventricular arrhythmias, 103
vertebrates, 137
vessels, 18, 143
viral infection, 125
viscosity, 17, 18, 29, 46
vision, 61

W

walking, 63, 64

water, 64, 145, 155
weakness, 28
white matter, 26, 28, 36
windows, 82, 113
withdrawal, 38, 90, 93, 94
Wnt signaling, 34
workers, 103
workload, 69
World Health Organization (WHO), 151
worldwide, x, 141, 142, 151
wound healing, 19

Y

yield, 127
young adults, 28, 120